What the Experts Say About
Food and Cancer

- Interviews with leading cancer researchers
- Why your current diet is a cancer time bomb
- The 7 foods and beverages that can dramatically lower your risk for common cancers

Rick Weissinger, MS, RD, LDN

2

Table of Contents

3

ACKNOWLEDGEMENTS

I would like to thank the many researchers who provided information used throughout this work. Each one patiently answered my questions, shared their discoveries, spent hours on the phone with me, and allowed me to tape our conversations in order to quote what they had to say.

In alphabetic order, these researchers include Dr. Vaqar Adhami; Dr. Rajesh Agarwal; Dr. Nihal Ahmad; Dr. R James Barnard; Dr. Phyllis Bowen; Dr. Andrew Collins; Dr. Alan Conney; Dr. Spiridione Garbisa; Dr. Andreas Gescher; Dr. Ed Giovannucci; Dr. David Jacobs; Dr. Andrew Joe; Dr. Coral LaMartiniere; Dr. Joseph Levy; Dr. Mohsen Meydani; Dr. Hasan Muhktar; Dr. Elizabeth Platz; Dr. Kedar Prasad; Dr. Cheryl Rock; Dr. Yoav Sharoni; Dr. Soraya Shirazi-Beechey; Dr. Shivendra Singh; Dr. Paul Talalay; Dr. Cynthia Thompson; Dr. Ivana Vucenik; Dr. I Bernard Weinstein; and Dr. Jin-Rong (Joseph) Zhou.

Special thanks to Dr. Fazlul Sarkar, for his generosity of spirit in giving to this work, his incredible talent as a researcher, and his dedication to cancer prevention.

This is for Anabelle

Introduction:
A New Approach to Understanding and Preventing Cancer

According to the American Cancer Society (ACS), nearly 1 of 2 American men and 1 of 3 American women develop some form of cancer. With these odds, we might think that cancer is unavoidable. However, most evidence confirms what health experts have been telling us for years; most cancers are preventable. As someone whose career has focused on promoting health, I have long wondered why our government and 'health care' system allocate so little time, effort, and money to preventing cancer and other lifestyle-related diseases.

My main reason for writing this work dovetailed with one of my long-standing professional goals, which is to make lofty-sounding but critically important scientific concepts understandable to the layman. This knowledge is desperately needed. In spite of the huge number of people affected by cancer, people seem to know little about the role of diet in its prevention. This seems to me a national tragedy of epic proportions. With respect to another major killer of Americans - that of cardiovascular disease - the public is aware that many preventable risk factors (elevated cholesterol, smoking) exist, and they can act on this knowledge if they so choose. However, we can't say the same for cancer prevention, because no one has done the work of explaining cancer growth to the public in ways they can understand. My aim in writing this work is simple. I want the average person to understand, if only at a basic level, how the foods they are eating, day in and day out, affects their cancer risk.

What *does* the average person know of these diseases? Studies have suggested that the public is misinformed about the real causes of most cancers (1) and considers these unavoidable. As one example, survey results published by the National Breast Cancer Coalition (NBCC) found that out of 1,000 women interviewed, 3 out of 4 felt they were "knowledgeable" about breast cancer. However, when the NBCC asked these women, "What is the most common risk factor for breast cancer?" more than half (56%) answered the question by stating that family history (i.e., 'bad genes') was to blame (2). This contrasts sharply with the evidence that genes influence only 5 to 10% of breast cancers. Cancer survivors are similarly uninformed; most attribute the cause of their cancer to factors beyond their control. Studies have also revealed that although many cancer patients make diet and lifestyle changes after they are diagnosed, most of them soon resume the same poor eating and exercise habits that increased their risk in the first place.

How do we know that developing healthy eating habits or changing our diets will pay off? The answer is, we have an *enormous* amount of evidence that says it does, of all different types. These studies include basic (laboratory) research; animal studies; epidemiological investigations; and clinical trials in humans. Epidemiological investigations often come first. For example, if a study of foods or nutrient intakes reveals that a population in the North part of a country (who eat a lot of rutabagas) has half the incidence of a cancer as those who live in the South (who hate rutabagas with a passion and never eat them), there is a good chance that there are some protective compounds in rutabagas that lower cancer risk. Laboratory research may follow in order to see which of these compounds inhibits cancer growth in cultures of cancer cells. If these studies show promise, animal studies are likely to follow, in which chemoprevention (cancer-preventive) and even therapeutic effects against many cancers may be demonstrated. However, clinical studies in humans at risk for cancer, or who are fighting an existing cancer, are considered to be the 'gold standard' of proof of an anti-malignancy effect. A typical study of this kind has involved giving a food or dietary supplement (lycopene, for example) to a group of patients who have (or are at risk for) cancer, while a similar group receives an identical looking 'dummy' pill (placebo). As it turns out, we already have evidence that, for example, soy foods, lycopene, green tea, resveratrol, curcumin, and an anti-cancer compound in whole grains and legumes (IP6) have cancer inhibiting effects in human populations, in the lab, in animals, and in humans fighting cancer. Given these tools, are we any closer to widespread cancer prevention?

The idea that we can prevent or treat a complex disease like cancer through the use of individual phytochemicals, vitamins, or minerals, separated from the foods nature put them in, sends the wrong message. For instance, if lycopene studies reveal an anti-cancer effect in humans, people may interpret these as saying: Why eat tomatoes, when we can just take a lycopene supplement? This has already happened with beta-carotene supplements, with no demonstrable benefit (and even an *increase* in cancer in the very persons at highest risk). On the other hand, if other studies fail to reveal an anti-cancer effect, the conclusion reached may be: don't waste your time eating foods that contain lycopene. Both messages are wrong, because they don't take into account an additive or synergistic effect of food components as a means of cancer prevention. Unhealthy diets turn on several 'switches' that spur cancer growth, and eating a limited number of foods that turn these switches off won't be helpful if other foods eaten at the same meal (or the next one) just flip these switches back on again. Or, as one researcher I interviewed put it, you'll have 'one foot on the brake, while the other is on the accelerator' of cancer growth.

In this manuscript, I've tried to explain the connections between diet and cancer risk by using metaphor and comparison, avoiding use of the technical language found in oncology journals. What you'll see summarized in these pages is evidence that the behind-the-scenes events determining cancer risk are more under your control than you might ever imagine. By the end of this book, you'll know to a great extent how and why cancers grow, how to use food to minimize your risk for getting cancer, and how to impede cancer growth if you're already fighting it.

An interesting feature of this manuscript is that it contains interviews with some of the world's leading investigators in diet and cancer, whose comments help to illustrate and emphasize certain critical points. Although this work differs from other books on this topic by virtue of its explanation of mechanisms and how diet impacts these, the conclusions are similar to what has been recommended by many cancer experts: diets composed mostly of plant foods should be emphasized for cancer prevention, along with a healthy weight and physically active lifestyle (3).

CHAPTER ONE

Next Stop, Cancerville: Why Everyone is on the Same Train

What would you say if you found out that you are being set up to develop cancer before you've even been born? No, there isn't an actual conspiracy of evil villains sitting around a boardroom table, James Bond-style, hatching plans for your early demise. However, both the food industry and our government *are* partly to blame for your cancer risk, because they have significant influences on the development of our eating habits. These habits affect the health of mothers and their unborn children (and in fact, our entire population) and as such, their importance can't possibly be taken too seriously.

The food industry exists, as most other industries do, to make a profit, and they do not feel any responsibility for your cancer risk. Our government, as was thoroughly detailed in Marion Nestle's *Food Politics*, is lobbied by the food industry to either say only nice things (or to keep silent) and/or to allow the purveyors of fast food and junk food to say what they want about their products. The food industry reduces the number of USDA inspectors at facilities that process beef, chicken, and other animal products; as a result, our meat supply is as polluted as the Hudson. They demand the right to advertise their products continually, and scream bloody murder if the government or public health advocates tries to restrict their right to 'free enterprise' or 'free speech'. In contrast, advertising of unhealthy foods is restricted in many other countries, as part of public health policy.

As a result, if you live in the U.S., you'll be programmed - brainwashed is just as good a word - to think that a Western diet is totally acceptable, even good for you. Your typical meals will contain generous amounts of animal protein, animal fat, sugar, and white flour. Even many of the snacks you eat between your meals will look like 'party' foods, devoid of fiber and the nutrients that whole, unprocessed foods provide. You'll experience what some scientists call a "one, two" hit: exposure to cancer-causing compounds found in these foods, and a low intake of essential nutrients and the plant-based food substances known as *phytochemicals* that help protect you against cancer.

By the age of 40, 50, 60 or 70, you will have eaten ten of thousands of meals like this, and the damage to your DNA will have resulted in the buildup of several mutations. Each of these gives future cancers the ability to survive in some way. Your chances will gradually grow extremely high that you'll be diagnosed with a common type: breast cancer, prostate cancer, colon cancer, lung cancer, skin cancer, or one of many others. If you've been a smoker, you probably won't be surprised at a cancer diagnosis; otherwise, you may never know what hit you, or why, because no one ever told you how cancer begins. "We have seen the enemy, and he is us," a slogan originally used on a poster for Earth Day in 1970, describes this state of affairs well. Most of us *are* our own worst enemy when it comes to cancer and other health problems, because we don't take healthy eating seriously.

Where it all begins: the origins of cancer

You don't have to be a scientist to know that pregnant women gain weight during pregnancy. If you've a keen observer, you may have noticed that women who gain too little weight during pregnancy often have smaller babies, while those who gain too much weight tend to have babies that are *bigger* than average. This extra growth is starting to look really important in cancer risk.

To understand why, you have to know what makes us grow. To start, you need lots of calories. Given that the importance of protein has been hyped to the heavens (more on this later) most people also know that protein foods are a must. Any Nutritionist worth their shingle will inform you that *both* calories and protein have to be well supplied, or growth will go nowhere. You can eat 5 times the protein you need, but none of it will make you grow if you don't have enough calories to *spare* that protein. Your body will simply break down the protein and use it to meet your energy needs. You may not get smaller, but you won't grow either.

When both calories and protein are plentiful, growth occurs. However, *over*growth often results when an *excess* of both are present. This has been the case since the start of the obesity epidemic in the U.S. Roughly 60% of women of childbearing age are either overweight or obese, and 15% to 20% of U.S. women are obese when they first become pregnant. Women who begin their pregnancy in an obese state have *eight times* the risk for having overweight babies as do women who are normal weight or simply 'overweight.' And the way we're gaining weight in the U.S. is beginning to look like we'll wind up resembling our super-obese descendants in the movie *Wall-E* (who, if you didn't see the movie, were amorphous blobs so heavy that that were no longer able to walk, and had to be levitated by machines).

Playing devil's advocate, some might say: Aren't fat babies more robust than small ones, and won't they eventually lose a lot of their body fat as they grow? The answers to these questions are complex, but looking past the immediate height and weight of an infant is important here. The problem is that dietary excesses have an impact on long-term 'programming' of the genes of these infants, and the program isn't always a good one. In the words of one group of researchers,

Recent epidemiological data link rapid growth in the womb to metabolic disease and obesity and also to breast and lung cancers.

In other words, overweight Moms who have overweight babies place them at higher risk for developing deadly diseases in adulthood, something that they would never knowingly do. As for why this occurs, scientists have concluded that exposing fetuses to diets rich in saturated fat and sugars affects levels of hormones and certain 'growth factors' involved in cancer risk. These have the ability to affect gene expression in utero, including cancer-causing genes ('oncogenes'). Proof that this occurs comes from studies that reveal a greater risk for breast cancer in women born at higher weights. If you are a woman who weighed more than 6.6 lbs. at birth, you are at higher risk; the highest risk for breast cancer – roughly 25% greater - occurs in women born weighing 8.8 lbs. or more (4000 grams).

Other than bodyweight, greater height is another indicator of being overfed. If you have any children or siblings with children, you've probably noticed that each generation has grown taller than the last. Parents tend to think this is a good thing; the data disagree. According to a multitude of studies, both childhood and adult tallness are related to higher risk for cancers of the breast, prostate, colon, rectum, endometrium, and blood forming system. Studies also suggest that obesity, exercise, diet and lifestyle during the many years between infancy and the finishing of growth in early adulthood are related to the development of cancers later in life. This tells us that there are opportunities to reduce cancer risk *in utero*, in childhood, and in adolescence.

The issue of weight gain during pregnancy is only one aspect of an individual's future cancer risk. *How* women become overweight – meaning, eating a lot of calorie dense, nutrient-poor foods – is yet another. The jury isn't in yet, but the evidence that's in shows that, by not eating healthier foods, women miss out on nutrients that are critical for controlling their child's future cancer risk. The risk for these childhood cancers (leukemia, neuroblastoma, and brain tumors) can be lowered, to some degree, by taking prenatal vitamins, but supplements don't completely remove the damage caused by excess weight gain and 'junk' diets.

If I've given the impression that women play the only role in their developing babies' cancer risk, let me clarify this. Semen quality in males has been found to play a role in childhood cancers, and both poor diet and smoking play roles here by damage the DNA in sperm.

You may, if your parents have raised you to eat differently and healthfully, enjoy a lower than average cancer risk. For the rest of America, the results are obvious. Cancer has become an epidemic that is far worse today than it was decades ago, when ex-President Richard Nixon declared a 'war on cancer' that was thought to be winnable within a few years. Although the cry is always for more research funding, I disagree. We know enough already about how cancer growth occurs to make a difference in peoples lives. It's time to share and teach this information.

The 'Nuts and Bolts' of Cancer

As one of my favorite authors once wrote, 'any significant event is *over-determined.*' Meaning, if it's a really meaningful event, it must have more than one cause. With cancer, the very high number of people affected implies it too is over-determined. Aside from over-nutrition, several other preventable steps, most of these related to your diet and lifestyle, occur over time to raise your risk. These events include: exposure to higher than normal blood levels of certain hormones and growth factors, damage to your DNA, combined with inadequate DNA repair; failure of budding tumor cells to experience a suicide-like process known as *apoptosis*; the acquired ability of cancer cells to spread (metastasize), involving a process known as *angiogenesis*; changes in your immune system that involve smoldering, low-level inflammation and inability to kill off rogue cells; increases in signals that allow cancer cells to divide; and a loss of the ability of these cells to keep from becoming cloned copies, a process known as *differentiation*.

Before I describe all these, let me begin the explanation of how the stage continues to be set throughout life for an eventual diagnosis of malignancy, through exposure to toxins and inadequate detoxification.

Toxin exposure, detoxification, and cancer risk

Carcinogenesis is a very prolonged process that may take 15 to 20 years. Many cells go in this direction, but the vast majority don't make it. During this silent period, *we have opportunities to interfere, block, or even reverse the damage that's being done.* The opportunities for prevention are many, but *they must go on during the entire life span.* [Italics mine]

- From an interview with Paul Talalay, M.D.
  John Jacob Abel Distinguished Service Professor of Pharmacology
  Director of the Laboratory for Molecular Sciences at Johns Hopkins
  University School of Medicine

'Toxins', or chemicals with potentially noxious effects, are a well-known cause of DNA damage and cancer. I'll list below some of the most common kinds of toxins you'll come in contact with, and then explain how healthier eating can help your body detoxify these poisons. Before I do, let me give you an idea of how obsessed people can be with the idea of detoxification. Use of the search engine GOOGLE recently yielded over fifteen *million* results, while the National Library of Medicine's website listed nearly 24,000 articles on detoxification. Considering that the number of results on the world-wide web outnumbered the scientific references by a factor of over 700 to 1, there is obviously a great deal of interest in this topic (and money to be made, besides), and the interest seems to be far greater in the public than in the scientific domain.

Speaking of making money: the somewhat less scientific consumer (layperson) view is one that invites being taken advantage of. Many consumers are, when it comes to detoxification, what the comedian W.C. Fields used to call the 'sucker born every minute.' We gladly give our hard-earned money to owners of high-end spas, who tell us that a buildup of toxins is the cause for our health problems, ranging from excess weight to morning brain fog. (Recently, I heard a well-known nutrition guru on a local public radio station, talking chapter and verse about his view that 'toxins' were the cause of most health problems, and of course selling products to 'cure' it. This contrasts sharply with the fact that chronic, low-grade inflammation is actually to blame for most diseases). The cure, we are often told, is one of a number of 'cleansing' regimes that typically include fasting, juices, herbs, body wraps, and sauna. If these aren't to your liking, you also have your choice of books on the subject, many of which don't contain scientific references to back up the text within. Almost without exception, these approaches promise eager granola-heads that they can rapidly detoxify their bodies, generally within a short period of days. Not only is the idea of eliminating decades of toxin buildup in a fraction of the time laughable; these 'quick fix' approaches also subtract from the legitimacy of what is otherwise a critical area of cancer prevention. Yet celebrities and the wealthy continue to flock to trendy retreats to partake of these treatments, with the illusion of attaining better health.

The more legitimate science of detoxification concerns itself with your body's ability to get rid of foreign compounds (for example, organic pollutants and inorganic heavy metals) or present in excess (medicines and hormones, for example). The underlying reason for our ability to perform these tasks is their essentiality for our survival as a species. Without our ability to get rid of these, a buildup of these substances would interfere with our health and reproduction. Thus we have evolved finely tuned bodily processes that function in tune with our food supply. And it functions quite well in most people, if we are given access to the nutrients found in health promoting foods that help these processes work.

Most chemical compounds that are associated with higher cancer risk are found in animal, not plant foods (see below). Although plants contain many natural pesticides (produced to keep insects and birds away), these obviously don't cause us harm, or they wouldn't be associated with *lower* cancer risk. Certain toxins found in meats pose an especially great risk for harm. (Funny how you never hear people complaining about these, although they will complain about the pesticide residues in fruits and vegetables!) These compounds include nitrosamines, dioxins, and *heterocyclic amines* (HCAs). I'll review these before getting to a discussion of how detoxification proceeds, and how your food choices affect these processes.

Nitrosamines and cancer risk

As a first example, let's consider the limits set on nitrates used as meat preservatives. Sodium nitrite was originally added to meats to maintain their color, and understandably so, because gray-looking meat isn't appetizing. The critics of synthetic preservatives may think of nitrates as toxic, but they are necessary. Without these, the lethal botulism toxin can form, so nitrites are clearly the lesser of two evils. However, when meat protein combines with nitrite, *nitrosamines* are formed. These are linked to several cancers, mainly the ones associated with the gut (stomach, colon, and rectum). Meat product manufacturers were probably *not* overjoyed at having their product associated with cancer. As a result, they've worked to reduce the amounts of nitrites in foods, or eliminated these altogether. Nevertheless, nitrosamines continue to be researched as a potential cause for certain cancers, including childhood brain tumors.

Dioxins and cancer risk

Dioxins are a general terms for a group of over 400 contaminants found everywhere in our environment. They are thought to be one of the most toxic man-made molecules, and are a by-product of industrial processes such as pesticide manufacturing and waste incineration. Interestingly (and tragically) dioxins are one of the toxins found in the dust that emergency workers inhaled after the bombing of the World Trade Center. They are also found in the herbicide known as Agent Orange, which was widely used during the Vietnam War. Not surprisingly, exposure to dioxin during the Vietnam War is associated with a greater risk of leukemia in Vietnam veterans, in addition to greater risk for prostate cancer.

The major sources of dioxin exposure in humans are animal products, especially milk, beef, poultry, pork, seafood, and even baby foods that contain meat. The International Food Information Council estimates that 95 percent of human exposure to dioxins comes from these foods. They also note that dioxin particles that fall from the air onto fruits and vegetables can be removed through washing. And if you're carrying extra poundage, take note: the Institute of Medicine (IOM) warns that getting these toxins out of your body becomes harder as you gain weight, because dioxins take up residence in body fat.

Some researchers have pointed to the fact that exposure to dioxins after industrial accidents doesn't always seem to increase cancer risk. Nevertheless, a publication by Germany's Federal Environmental Agency that looked at the exposure limits set by different countries revealed that it's very hard to set restrictions on dioxins, given we only have animal studies to go on. However, it's troubling that infants are the group most highly exposed to these poisons, whose intake is at least *ten times* as much as adults.

Environmental chemicals and cancer risk

In 2009, a paper was published in a medical journal by a group of scientists, researchers, and clinicians representing the opinion of a scientific organization known as the Endocrine Society. This paper summarized the data linking a specific group of environmental chemicals ('endocrine disruptors,' defined as "agent(s) that interferes with synthesis, secretion, transport, metabolism, binding action, or elimination of natural blood-borne hormones") to the risk for cancer and diseases related to cancer (early puberty, obesity, and diabetes). Dioxins are among these.

The Society came to the conclusion that endocrine-disrupting chemicals represent a significant potential risk in terms of certain human cancers. Although most data come from studies in test tubes or small animals and are hard to translate to humans, there appears to be good reason to avoid polychlorinated biphenyls (PCBs), polybrominated biphenyls (PBBs), plastics [bisphenol A (BPA)], plasticizers (phthalates), pesticides [methoxychlor, chlorpyrifos, fungicides (vinclozolin), and dichlorodiphenyltrichloroethane (DDT)]. But how can an average person keep their exposure low, without a degree in toxicology to help them spot where these toxins exist?

Toxins in cooked meats – a good reason to make barbecuing a 'rare' occasion

In addition to the nitrosamines and dioxins, there are other toxins in meat that might make you want to choose meat substitutes more often. In this case, it's how meat gets cooked, and there's an interesting story behind it.

Roughly 30 years ago (so the story goes) a Japanese scientist was on holiday with his wife when he smelled smoke coming from their kitchen. Knowing that *cigarette* smoke contained cancer-causing substances got him thinking: Is it possible that smoke from the burning of *foods* might be another source of toxins? This led to the finding that meats cooked at high temperatures (barbecuing, broiling, roasting) contain DNA-mutating *heterocyclic amines* (HCAs). The way many of us wind up getting most of our HCAs is from good old-fashioned barbecuing. During this process, meat fat is burned on hot coal or wood, and the smoke carries HCAs up and onto the meat. In this way, even lower fat meat like chicken can, simply due to the way it's cooked, provide a cancer risk similar to red meat.

HCAs are thought to be one of the reasons that eating well-done meat is linked to a higher risk for cancers of the breast, colon/rectum, prostate, and pancreas. In fact, eating as little as 10 grams per day (one-third of an ounce) of well-done meat has been linked to prostate cancer, compared to men who did not eat meat prepared this way. Cooking your meat only until rare or medium can help keep HCAs from accumulating in foods. However, doing so may increase your risk for food poisoning. Neither is an attractive outcome.

Turkey burgers begin to sound better than hamburger when we consider that people who more often eat high fat meats have a higher risk for cancers of the colon, lung, prostate, and blood (lymphoma). However, other toxins appear in meats when they are cooked; one of these belongs to a class called 'advanced glycation end products' (AGEs, or *glycotoxins*). AGEs are very strongly proinflammatory. Given that chronic, low level inflammation is known to contribute to cancer risk (more on this in just a while), stick to veggie burgers (or make barbecued meats something you eat only on special occasions) if you want to keep your cancer risk low. (Believe me when I tell you that as you eat these less often, the enjoyment you obtain increases).

These are only a few of the many toxins our bodies have to process. Many scientists believe that, because many of us live in or near large metropolitan areas and manufacturing plants, we exists in a virtual 'sea of chemicals' in which our exposure is continuously higher each year. Although advocating for tighter environmental regulations can help control these exposures, corporations often find ways to evade these. Taking care of your inner environment, on the other hand, is something you *can* control.

How your body gets rid of toxins: Biotransformation and 'Phase I' detoxification

The human body has systems for both limiting our exposure to toxins and for getting rid of these. Your gut is the first barrier, and works by getting rid of toxins in the stool. The kidneys also get a turn; they help excrete toxins that have been made water-soluble by passing these out in urine. However, another detoxification process that involves changing a chemical's structure is a key aspect of cancer prevention. This process, known as *biotransformation*, is the single most important defense against chemicals because it gets these ready for removal from the body. Biotransformation is also a process in which diet and phytochemicals especially play important roles, which I'll describe below. The human liver is what does the bulk of the job, although your skin, your gut, and your lungs also have a role in detoxification. This system uses enzymes that first activate and then inactivate these toxins, both of which are necessary for their elimination. Everything foreign - drugs, food preservatives, food dyes, herbicides, and chemicals you ingested or inhaled over the past day – is a target for this system.

The first step in processing toxins involves the work of 'Phase I' (cytochrome P450 or CYP450) enzymes. These proteins work by first making toxins more water-soluble, which helps the kidney do the work of excretion. Yet by doing so, the CYP450 system converts non-reactive chemicals to potential carcinogens. Although this is coupled with other (Phase II) reactions that get rid of them for good, in some persons (ones with different CYP450 genes), an excess activity of these toxin-activating enzymes may occur. This might be considered dangerous, but it appears to be a response to the load of toxins (for example, in a smoker) that a person is dealing with.

I interviewed Dr. Alan Conney, a Rutgers University expert on detoxification processes, to understand this process more clearly. "It's not *always* the case that increasing Phase I enzymes is a bad thing," Dr. Conney confirmed. "In some situations, it may be a good thing. For instance, treating the skin of certain animals with Phase I inducers inhibits the cancer-causing ability of known skin carcinogens. If we didn't have Phase I enzymes, the chemicals that we're exposed to would stay in the body for close to a lifetime, which would probably result in some kind of toxicity," offered Dr. Conney. "We would probably not survive without them."

Often, people are prescribed medicines that (like all drugs) must be processed by Phase I enzymes. These include those that lower cholesterol, blood pressure, blood sugar, inflammation, treat allergy symptoms, and others. Many of these come with warnings to not drink grapefruit juice, which by inhibiting Phase I enzymes can allow drugs to build up to potentially dangerous levels. (You can imagine how the citrus growers of Florida, California, and Texas reacted to this news. After hurricanes and tornadoes battered Florida's citrus crop, prices went up; however, this made sales go down, and grapefruit juice sales decreased twice as much as orange juice sales between 2003 and 2007.)

Phase II detoxification

Of the two main ways your body handles toxins, the Phase II enzymes may be more important. One reason is that Phase II enzymes have antioxidant effects. These help lower your cancer risk by neutralizing DNA-damaging free radicals. Not surprisingly, higher levels of Phase II enzymes are linked to a lower risk for chemically induced cancers. These enzymes work by hooking up water-soluble, Phase I-activated toxins to other chemicals that act as chaperones, which escort these out of your body.

The importance of Phase II enzymes to cancer prevention is not in doubt. However, each of us is, based on the genes we get from our parents, different with regard to how active these enzymes are. For example, having a 'null' (inactive) version of the gene for one particular Phase II enzyme (GST) is associated with a higher risk for cancers of the lung, larynx, bladder, and for certain brain tumors. In another scenario, people who have lower levels of GST in the colon have a greater risk for colon cancer.

The most exciting news about Phase II enzymes is that although we don't have the ability to change how our genes influence these, we may not need to. Through making certain changes in our diets, we have a degree of control over them, and can induce these enzymes to work harder at lowering our cancer risk. Even in people with lower levels of these enzymes, eating more *cruciferous* vegetables (broccoli, cauliflower, cabbage, Brussels sprouts) or *Allium* vegetables (onion and garlic) raises activity of the Phase II system. In smokers who are missing one of these protective detox enzymes, eating more cruciferous vegetables appears to result in a lower risk for lung cancer, compared with smokers who don't eat these vegetables as often. Although evidence is lacking, there are reasons to believe that you might get the same benefit if you're exposed to second-hand smoke too. As might be expected, your cancer risk may be lower if you're lucky enough to have Phase II enzymes in good working condition *and* you eat foods that make these enzymes work harder. As one example, if you happen to be a guy who has well-functioning Phase II enzymes (in this case, GSTM-1) and you eat more broccoli, cabbage, and cauliflower than most men, you might be at the lowest risk for prostate cancer, compared to those men without the gene or with low intake of cruciferous vegetables.

Nutrition professionals, as well as many health-conscious consumers, already know that the cruciferous vegetables are important for ramping up Phase II enzymes. However, there are other phytochemicals in plant foods that help with detoxification, and they lower cancer risk in several other ways. I'll turn to some of these now, starting by introducing you to a novel concept: the existence of a suicide program called *apoptosis* (pronounced 'ay poe toe sis') that somehow goes wrong in cancer cells, and how you can use your diet to right that wrong.

The Science of Self-Destruction: Getting Cancers to Implode

If you knew you had the power to make cancer cells growing in your body self-destruct, would you want to learn how? Hopefully, you believe the answer here is a no-brainer, so we can proceed as if your answer is an enthusiastic, "Of course!"

If you're game, let me give you a view of the possibility that you don't need an Oncologist to kill your cancer cells, because you get them to kill themselves. This process is known as *apoptosis*, and is a major goal of both cancer prevention *and* treatment. With a continued understanding of what factors would enable average people to trigger apoptosis, we might be able to make cancer prevention something most people can achieve at home. We might also consider it a *pro*active stance we can take against cancer, rather than the *re*active one taken by most people, who do little until they are given the bad news.

Normally, apoptosis occurs in your body's cells if they're virus-infected, old, or damaged. Apoptosis differs from another type of cell death called *necrosis*, which can occur from physical injury, damage from infection, or chemical poisoning. Necrotic cell death is a messy, violent form of cell death that causes inflammation, which can further drive cancer growth. By contrast, apoptosis is neater. It involves breakdown of a cancer cell's internal cell structure in a piece-by-piece fashion, a gradual loss of its shape, and eventually shrinking down to near nothingness, followed by cannibalization by your white blood cells.

Dr. Andreas Gescher, a Professor of Biochemical Toxicology in the Department of Cancer Studies at the UK's University of Leicester, described apoptosis when we spoke about his work with the phytochemical *resveratrol* (found in large amounts in red wine, but also in grapes and peanuts). "Cancer is a disease in which cells lose the ability to undergo the normal dying process," he explained. "These malignant cells have developed some very elegant and clever ways to avoid this process. My coworkers and I, and many other scientists who work in cancer prevention or treatment, have been trying to developing ways in which cancer cells can regain the ability for apoptosis."

Why do cancer cells lose this crucial ability to kill themselves off? The answers are still being debated, but diet plays a role. In this section, I'll explain how excesses of both calories and animal protein prevent apoptosis. I'll also detail how eating more phytochemical-containing foods can reverse this process, and increase your body's production of protein-munching enzymes (*caspases*) that activate apoptosis.

Too much food, too few suicidal cancer cells

Animal research on restriction of excess food intake has revealed what experts have been saying for many years about obesity and cancer risk: apoptosis can occur by cutting back food intake by as little as 10%. In these studies, monkeys given less food had lower cancer rates and (surprisingly) less muscle loss than animals given more food. Human studies are showing similar benefits, according to a number of experts I interviewed. One of these, Dr. R. James Barnard, a UCLA scientist and Director of Research at the Pritikin Longevity Center, has done research on the effects of diet and exercise on prostate cancer. Dr. Barnard's work involves a protein called *insulin-like growth factor* (IGF-1) known to promote cancer growth.

"IGF-1 is a known stimulant for cancer cell growth that inhibits apoptosis," he began. "We've shown in men who we've placed on a very low fat diet and regular daily exercise that IGF-1 levels drop dramatically. We've also been able to show that, at the same time, IGF binding proteins increase, leaving less IGF free to promote growth of tumor cells."

Dr. Hasan Mukhtar, a Professor of Cancer Research at the University of Wisconsin's Medical School, also commented on the link between IGF and prostate cancer when we spoke about his research on green tea. "What we call the 'IGF axis' - IGF-1 and its binding proteins - are imbalanced in patients with prostate cancer," he explained. "It may be that the same way that people with diabetes are advised to eat a certain way to bring their blood sugar back down to normal limits, we will be advising people to use foods that decrease their IGF levels to lower cancer risk," he continued. "We are advocating that the IGF axis could be used as a measure to determine the effectiveness of cancer prevention methods in humans."

The IGF axis Dr. Mukhtar spoke of can be affected by what you eat, your weight, and by how much you exercise. While under-nutrition will cause a lack of growth factors like IGF, eating enough to maintain a healthy weight will allow for a more-or-less normal production. If we eat too much and gain excess weight, we may produce more growth factors. Combining eating just enough to maintain a healthy weight with exercise accomplishes two important aims: it keeps IGF-1 levels in a normal range, and it increases proteins that tie up IGF (IGF binding proteins, IGFBPs) so that it can't exert an effect on cancer cells. IGFBP-3, which binds up most IGF-1, may also prevent cancer cell growth directly by triggering apoptosis. And people who are fighting an existing cancer need to be aware of how diet can affect this growth factor too; IGF-1 plays an important role in promoting resistance to chemotherapy and radiation. Because IGF-1 is influenced by diet (see below), this has enormous implications for diet during cancer therapy.

'Access to excess' is an important influence on the IGF axis. In one study that neatly showed the effect of food intake on IGF-1 levels, scientists looked at two genetically similar groups of East Indians. One of these groups remained in India and ate a traditional vegetarian diet, while the other moved to the U.K. and soon began eating a diet that provided more calories and meat. As suspected, IGF-1 levels increased and IGF binding proteins decreased in the migrant group who were eating more calories and animal protein. There have been several other studies that compared cancer risk between people living in their native homelands (and eating traditional diets) with people in the same ethnic group that moved to the U.S. Practically all these found higher cancer risk within one generation of eating a Western diet and living inactive lifestyles.

IGF-1 increases when insulin does, and insulin increases when we gain weight. It stands to reason then that the foods that have the greatest impact on post-meal insulin (starchy carbohydrates like bread, rice, macaroni, and fruits) *should* represent a higher cancer risk, because their effect on insulin *should* increase IGF-1 more than other foods. If that were so, cancer rates should increase when we eat more carbs. But that's not what happens. Carbs are generally *not* linked to IGF-1 levels, and the traditional diets eaten in non-Westernized countries that are carb-rich are known to protect against, not raise, cancer risk.

So if a high intake of carbohydrates doesn't excessively raise IGF-1, what does? The answer is SAD – the Standard American Diet, otherwise known as a 'Western' diet. The SAD diet provides an excess of calories, saturated fat, cholesterol, and animal protein – the nutrient with the greatest impact on IGF-1. Clinical studies have that found IGF-1 levels are stimulated by drinking milk; no surprise, since this is what it is supposed to do for growing calves. IGF-1 also increases as protein increases from 'normal' amounts recommended by nutrition experts to the excess levels (one and one-half to twice the recommended amount) which many Americans eat every day. Importantly, a high intake of animal protein raises IGF-1 more than plant sources of protein (like beans, nuts, or grains) or other food groups do. And while soy protein *does* cause an increase in IGF-1 similar to animal protein, it also increases IGF binding proteins, which makes it both a high-quality, growth-promoting protein *and* one that is better for cancer prevention.

Dairy, animal protein, and growth: a cancer-causing myth?

Let's examine the relationship between dairy products, IGF-1 levels, and cancers related to IGF-1's effects a little closer. Americans have been told for decades by the dairy industry and many government agencies that we need to drink milk and eat other growth-promoting animal foods every day of our lives if we want to be healthy. This myth, one among many addressed in a scary but enlightening fashion by Dr. Marion Nestle in *Food Politics: How the Food Industry Influences Nutrition and Health*, may be the single greatest cause of cancer (and of the health care crisis in general) that's developed over the past decades. One example of this kind of programming is the idea that children should drink milk several times each day to get enough protein and calcium. Parents encourage this, because they know that the protein and calcium in milk help with bone growth, an effect that makes children grow taller. However, the price these children pay for the increased height may not be worth it. Greater height has been linked with higher risk for breast cancer, ovarian cancer, certain blood cancers, pancreatic cancer, and prostate cancer. Many animal proteins that raise IGF-1 are also high in fat (eggs, whole milk, and beef, for example). Higher total fat intake is associated with lower levels of IGF binding proteins. This is no doubt among the reasons that eating too much fat has been linked to greater risk for certain cancers.

One giant step to lower IGF-1-related cancers: slim down

People eating lower-calorie diets can decrease their IGF-1 levels over 30%, compared to people eating much higher calorie Western diets. Being overweight is tied to inflammation, and to higher insulin output, both of which suppress apoptosis. So if losing weight normalizes growth factors and apoptosis, which kinds of calories should be cut first?

Most experts agree that the so-called 'empty' calories (from soda, fruit drinks, and junk foods) should be the first calories you should cut down on. After all, even many high-cholesterol foods provide essential nutrients. If eaten only occasionally and in small amounts, they can add variety and important vitamins and minerals (vitamins B6, B12, iron, zinc, selenium etc.). By contrast, simple sugars provide only calories. After sugars, cutting back on animal protein seems wise, for several reasons. First, experts in protein nutrition have found that the need for protein in healthy, stable persons doesn't exceed 15% of calories, and according to the World Health Organization, even 5% of calories is adequate, given enough protein-sparing calories. (Protein needs are however somewhat higher in persons who are in a growth phase or recovering from surgery or wounds). This should make protein the very last nutrient we consider when you deciding what to eat, way below even the type of fat you use. Animal protein is also the main source of saturated fat and cholesterol in our diets. Although you may think this matters only if you're avoiding heart disease, think again: many cancer cells depend on a surplus of cholesterol at a certain point in their development. Making cholesterol less unavailable can trigger apoptosis, so cutting way back on red meat, cheese, eggs, whole milk, butter, and other animal foods high in animal fat and protein should be your next step. There are at least three other ways you'll lower your cancer risk from making this diet change. The first is removing dioxins from your diet; the second is reducing your body's production of excess hormones involved in cancer risk (see Chapter Eight - The Grain Gain: How Whole Grains Fight Cancer). The third benefit is making room in your diet for the 'healthy' fats (nuts, seeds, and cooking oils high in unsaturated fat) that can lower your cancer risk by reducing inflammation and by providing phytochemicals and critically important fat-soluble nutrients like vitamins E and K.

If you think cutting back on saturated fat and cholesterol means depriving yourself of good, healthy, tasty foods, think again. While eating mainly plant foods can help lower IGF-1, you can still indulge in your favorite foods on special occasions (birthdays, national holidays). Dr. Barnard commented that even the Pritikin center, which has always served a low fat, high fiber, vegetarian diet, has been serving more fish. With respect to diet and IGF-1, he maintains, "You can still eat a lot of low-calorie, high-carbohydrate foods [fruits, vegetables, potatoes, rice, and cereals] that are very filling, and you don't have to walk around hungry all the time. The flip side of the typical Western diet is that you're not only affecting the IGF system. You're submitting the body to a tremendous array of phytochemicals and antioxidants that should reduce the risk for all kinds of cancer."

Exercise also affects the IGF axis. When your muscles work, they need less insulin to use blood sugar. As you increase your exercise and burn calories without insulin, your body produces less of this hormone, and IGF-1 levels decrease. For example, runners in one study had levels that were 12% lower than sedentary people. Exercise also increases IGF binding proteins. In a mega-study of more than 41,000 Australians, the most active persons had the highest levels of IGF binding proteins, and were almost 50% less likely to die from colorectal cancer.

For some of us, combining *both* changes in our eating and exercise habits is needed to affect the IGF axis and cancer risk. Dr. Barnard and his co-workers observed the effect on prostate cancer when men in their study attempted to change diet alone or in combination with exercise. "Men just doing exercise for an hour per day got substantial results, but not as good as those that were on the diet *and* exercise program," he confirmed. The results obtained from a combination of a vegan diet and exercise program were at first only reductions in prostate-specific antigen (PSA, a marker of prostate cancer growth). However, after two years on this regimen, results were more meaningful. Of the 43 men eating the vegan diet and exercising, only 2 (5%) needed medical therapy. "The majority of them so far haven't needed more aggressive treatment (radiation, surgery) of their prostate cancer," Dr. Barnard added. By comparison, 13 out of 49 men (27%) in the group not following the vegan diet/exercise plan needed medical or surgical treatment for increased prostate cancer growth.

Several other foods have the ability to affect apoptosis (and can lower your cancer risk in other ways besides). They include soy foods, green tea, lycopene, cruciferous vegetables, garlic, and resveratrol, and I'll discuss these in later chapters. These same phytochemicals also affect another key process in cancer growth that allows tumors to change in size from a non-threatening toaster crumb to an army that can take you over entirely. This process is called *angiogenesis*.

Angiogenesis: A chemical vampire that spreads cancer

Imagine two women from two different cities awakening miles apart one morning. Both follow the same monthly ritual by performing breast self-examination. While doing so, both find a lump and are concerned enough to see a physician. After a series of tests, these women are diagnosed with breast cancer. One is told that her tumor is localized, that it can be surgically removed, and that she has a good chance for a full recovery. The second woman is told that the cancer has spread, that she will need extensive treatment, and that her chances of survival beyond five years aren't good.

The situation that the second woman finds herself is in is all too common, because most cancers are caught *after* they have fully developed, rather than in an earlier phase. The critical difference between the two is that the second woman's cancer has undergone a preventable step called *angiogenesis*. This process allows a malignant tumor to metastasize (spread to other parts of the body). When cancers enter into this phase, chances for survival drop dramatically.

When I think about angiogenesis, I picture microscopic cancer cells with little fangs, sucking on a blood vessel like a tiny vampire. Although the description is a crude one, the reality is that budding tumors *do* use their host's blood supply to obtain the nourishment they need to grow, much as a vampire needs the blood of the living to survive.

The late surgeon and cancer researcher Dr. Judah Folkman spent half his 72 years proving that angiogenesis is crucial for cancer growth, and he deserves nearly all the credit for this discovery. However, many other scientists have done critically important work that links angiogenesis with diet and cancer prevention, which is critical to prevent the development of a full-blown malignancy. Let's start with an explanation of what angiogenesis is, and why it's so important.

Simply put, angiogenesis is the creation of new blood vessels. If you've got a heart muscle that has its blood supply blocked with cholesterol deposits, angiogenesis is literally life saving. However, if you've got a growing cancer, angiogenesis can be a death sentence. Access to blood vessels are critical for tumors, because they provide nutrient-rich blood cancers needs for growth. Without this blood supply, a tumor can't exceed 1 cubic millimeter – about the size of a toaster crumb. If tumors remained this size, they wouldn't be a serious threat, and if discovered, they could be easily (surgically) removed or killed by radiation. In fact, there's evidence from autopsy studies of cancers being found in people who never reported having symptoms while living. The extent of these undetected cancers is actually quite remarkable; researchers have estimated that 1 in 3 men have evidence of prostate cancer when they die. However, most of these tumors are so small that they're considered not worthy of treating. How can so many men appear healthy and without any signs and symptoms, even though they have a cancerous tumor? Suppression by the immune system is one possibility (more on this topic in just a while). However, the more likely reason these tumors don't metastasize and become full-blown cancers is that they haven't undergone a critical process called the 'angiogenic switch.' The importance of this process for tumor development was described in an article written by Dr. Folkman and his colleagues from Harvard Medical School's Department of Surgery:

Tumor progression depends on sequential events, including a switch to the angiogenic phenotype (i.e., initial recruitment of blood vessels). Failure of a microscopic tumor to complete one or more early steps in this process may lead to delayed clinical manifestation of the cancer. *Microscopic human cancers can remain in an asymptomatic, non-detectable, and occult state for the life of a person.* (Italics mine)

If you pause for a few moments and think about it, the concept that you can actually *have* a cancer without experiencing the *illness* that goes with it is mind-boggling. What these scientists are actually saying is that although you might not be able to prevent the creation of cancerous cells, suppressing angiogenesis may prevent these from becoming life-threatening tumors. Limiting angiogenesis after a tumor is already established is also considered an important part of cancer treatment, because it can halt tumor growth and stabilize disease progression. However, this doesn't necessarily lead to a cure, so from a preventive standpoint, stopping angiogenesis before it starts seems a better strategy.

Growth factors grow you - and cancers too

Angiogenesis doesn't occur without a trigger, and one of these includes growth factors. As we discussed above, certain growth factors are relevant to cancer by opposing apoptosis. Others are more central to angiogenesis, but it's more than likely they all work together. These include *vascular endothelial growth factor* (VEGF), a growth factor that triggers the 'angiogenic switch' in cancer metastasis. VEGF works like a construction foreman, helping construct new 'pipelines' (blood vessels) from the tumor to the bloodstream.

Your body can't make a significant amount of growth factors without having enough energy on board, but if there's one thing Americans have in abundance, it's energy, stored as body fat. Your excess body fat actually produces VEGF, which explains a lot of the connection between our current twin epidemics of obesity and cancer.

I spoke with Dr. Elizabeth Platz, an Epidemiologist with the Johns Hopkins Bloomberg School of Public Health, regarding her studies on the relationships between calorie intake, exercise output, growth factors and cancer risk. "We believe that overeating, under-exercising, and excess weight gain lead to changes in growth factors that increase angiogenesis," she explained. "We've seen prostate cancer incidence increase in some Asian populations within the same generation when they changed their lifestyle by eating more, being less active, and gaining weight."

Excess body fat increases other growth factors involved in cancer, including *hepatocyte growth factor* (HGF). HGF is produced in excess in women with breast cancer, and is linked with greater likelihood of breast cancer death. The links between HGF, body fat, and breast cancer also explain findings dating back over 30 years of greater risk for breast cancer in overweight, post-menopausal women. Researchers have long suspected, and have recently confirmed, that being overweight at the time of breast cancer diagnosis decreases chances for survival.

The green light on angiogenesis needs more than just growth factors, however. There are two other influences on this process worth mentioning, because they are diet-related and under your control to some degree. The first is inflammation, which enables angiogenesis by making your immune system produce growth factors. Inflammation drives cancer growth in many other ways, including increasing production of something called hypoxia-inducible factor (HIF) that has a key role in angiogenesis. The second influence on angiogenesis involves protein-digesting enzymes (metalloproteinases, MMPs). MMPs break down the walls between tissues that would normally separate tumors from healthy, non-cancerous tissues. As such, MMPs are a key feature of metastatic cancer and an important target of cancer therapy.

In later chapters, I'll detail how phytochemicals in foods we eat interfere with the processes that allow angiogenesis. Coming up, I'll review what the science says about some other types of growth-promoting agents - your hormones – and how they affect your cancer risk.

Cancer risk in the 21st century: hormonally yours

For many of us, the word 'hormones' might trigger thoughts and memories of puberty, mood swings, and menopause. The majority of Americans don't equate hormones with cancer. Yet an excess of certain hormones is a key reason why clinical cancer specialists are seeing more patients over the past couple of decades than they previously did.

If we are diagnosed with a hormone-related problem, we naturally think of seeing a hormone specialist (an Endocrinologist). This is of course the right move, because there may be something seriously wrong. However, millions of Americans have sub-clinical issues with hormones that don't imply overt disease and are below the diagnostic radar. These are problematic for two reasons: first, because they are still high enough to raise our cancer risk over the long term, and second, because they are the result of our lifestyle, a fact of which the great majority of us are not informed.

This concept might be troubling to many people because, in general, we don't tend to think of hormones as something we can control. The very idea that diet could affect your hormone levels seems strange. However, diet is often a cause of hormone-related problems that can often be changed without medical help. For men, testosterone is the hormone involved in prostate cancer risk; for women, high estrogen levels are a risk factor for cancers of the breast and reproductive organs. To get a good idea of why the hormone-cancer link is so critical, consider that *roughly 65% of all cancers are hormonally related.* Anti-hormone treatments – not chemotherapy or radiation - are also considered the state-of-the-art for most breast cancers and for the more aggressive kind of prostate cancer.

In this section, I'll explain why greater hormone exposure raises your risk for these more common types of cancer. I'll also explain how diet can impact hormone levels. In later chapters, I'll describe how eating certain phytochemical containing foods can reduce your risk for these hormone related cancers.

Why more hormones = more cancer

As any adolescent or parent of a teen knows, hormones make things grow. They're supposed to, at a certain age, when they take a quantum leap and increase to blood levels the body hadn't yet been exposed to. However, when they remain elevated, there's cause for concern.

Dr. Cheryl Rock, a Professor of Family and Preventive Medicine at the University of California at San Diego, described the effects of hormones as cancer growth factors during a discussion we had about her work on diet and cancer risk. "Hormones are chemical signals; they're like a letter in the mail that gets sent from one place, like the ovaries or body fat where estrogen is made, and gets picked up by another, like the breast or endometrial lining of the uterus," she began. "The importance of these hormones is that cancer is a process in which growth is no longer well-regulated. There are *some* tissues that are more sensitive to these growth factors than others, and estrogen has a more stimulating effect in breast tissue than in some other part of the body," she continued.

Girls are a better example of the effects of hormone excess than are boys, because they start to make larger amounts of estrogen when body fat reaches a certain level (usually after age 12 or 13, but earlier if kids are over-fed; more on this point in just a bit). Estrogen acts as a signal in breast cells, turning on growth of breast tissue. This is fine and well and there'd be major cause for concern if this process *didn't* happen, because it would imply disease. The problem with estrogen exposure for girls is one of excess, and one that starts with being overfed.

The root of this problem is the current epidemic of pediatric obesity, which causes body fat accumulation at an earlier age then ever before. Having more body fat converts testosterone to estrogen, so girls are exposed to a higher amount of the main female hormone at a younger age. Puberty begins as a result, and so does breast cancer risk, which depends in part on *total lifetime* exposure to estrogens. Early puberty not only increases the risk for breast cancer; it decreases breast cancer *survival* in women who start having periods at or before age eleven. Delayed menopause, another indicator of a greater lifetime estrogen exposure, also elevates breast cancer risk. By comparison and in other (non-Western) cultures where child obesity is less common, women have a lower risk for breast cancer. "One of the reasons that Asian women have a lower breast cancer risk is that they start their periods much later, so their total lifetime exposure to reproductive hormones is much less," confirmed Dr. Rock. Even this advantage is being eroded quickly, as Western eating habits have spread to Asian countries and created an epidemic of child obesity.

Hormone overload and cancer: an ignored national crisis

A 1997 study from the University of North Carolina's Department of Maternal and Child Health that involved more than 17,000 girls found evidence that young girls are being exposed to a high degree of hormone overload. By 8 years of age, over 48% of African-American girls and nearly 15% of white girls had begun physical development of secondary sexual characteristics, including breast growth, not usually seen until at least age 11 or 12. According to these researchers,

> *These data suggest that girls seen in a sample of pediatric practices from across the United States are developing pubertal characteristics at younger ages than currently used norms.*

Dr. John McDougall, a Physician who uses plant-based diets in his medical practice, points out that the age at which girls start maturing (menarche) has decreased significantly over time in most developed countries. As an example, Dr. McDougall pointed out that menarche was uncommon in women of Papua New Guinea in the 1960's before 18 to 19 years of age, due to the fact that these people ate a nearly vegetarian, very low-fat diet. It's unlikely that girls living in the United States will change to such a diet. However, the kind of diet most kids are eating here in the U.S. is causing not only hormone imbalances; it's increasing obesity and diabetes, which are also linked with higher cancer risk. Over-nourished adolescent boys may suffer the same increase in cancer risk as girls, thanks to evidence linking certain indicators of overnutrition (high birth weight and greater adult height) with an increased risk of the more aggressive type of prostate cancer.

Other than the hormones involved in sexual maturation and reproduction, one of the body's better-known hormones is also involved in cancer risk. Like estrogen and testosterone, it appears in gross excess before you begin to get ill from its effects. Yet you need this hormone every second of every day, and without it you couldn't derive the energy you need to keep your body running. This hormone is insulin.

Insulin and cancer risk

When we think of hormones, we tend to think of gender and reproduction, not blood sugar. Yet insulin is known as a 'classic' hormone, one needed to use sugar and other nutrients. Insulin also has a role as a growth factor that contributes to cancer risk. The question is, how might you know if you are in a high-risk group that makes too much insulin?

To answer this question, we should do what we did with estrogen: look for people who may have the greatest exposure to this hormone. They aren't hard to find; they're usually the ones who weigh the most. Scientists estimate that between 3% and 16% of the U.S. population are resistant to the effects of insulin and over-produce this hormone. Insulin resistance is at the root of 'metabolic syndrome,' a cluster of symptoms involving elevation in blood sugar, blood pressure, blood fats, obesity, inflammation, and other abnormalities that increase the risk for heart attack and stroke. This syndrome is estimated to affect more than one-third of all adults and up to 50% of elderly, and significantly increases your cancer risk.

UCLA Physiologist RJ Barnard detailed several roles for excess insulin in cancer risk during our interview. As it turns out, insulin works with in cooperation with other hormones in ways than increase cancer risk. He pointed out that as the amount of insulin our bodies make increases, the amount of sex hormone binding globulins (SHBG) declines. This leaves more estrogen and testosterone available to grow hormone-dependent cancers. Insulin also increases both the production of estrogen by fat cells and IGF-1. This 'hormonal cascade' explains in part (though not entirely) how the rise in cancer tagged along with the obesity epidemic in the U.S.

Associations between high blood insulin levels (hyperinsulinemia) and cancer risk also show up in human population studies. Hyperinsulinemia has been linked to greater risk for breast cancer, colorectal cancer, endometrial cancer, liver cancer, and mortality from prostate cancer. Many of these studies link hyperinsulinemia with excess body fat and elevated hormone levels in ways that make it hard to separate the cancer-promoting effects of one over another. Although smoking, poor magnesium intake, and genetics can all contribute to insulin resistance, it's obvious that being overweight is what causes this syndrome in most people. Obesity raises cancer risk in ways other than hormone excess; it also does so by increasing inflammation through your immune system. Chronic, low-grade inflammation ensues and continues over a period of years, contributing to cancer risk through DNA damage and other pathways.

Bodyweight and hormone levels: why losing excess weight lowers cancer risk

Being overweight (fat, not muscle) was, not too long ago, thought of as unsightly, but not dangerous. The problem is one of context, and the context in the U.S. is being overweight, inactive, *and* eating a relatively toxic diet. Limiting our discussion to just having excess body fat, the cancer risk comes from the evidence that this fat, particularly fat stored on the abdomen, acts like a chemical factory, churning out several kinds of hormones and hormone-like chemicals that can increase cancer growth. For example, being overweight causes a woman to produce more estrogen. Body fat also produces other hormones (including leptin and prolactin) and hormone-like chemicals (interleukins and growth factors) that can increase cancer growth.

"Hormone secretion and activity is influenced a lot by energy balance and obesity, regardless of whether you're eating too much protein, carbohydrate, or fat," Dr. Rock confirmed. "When a woman gets overweight - especially an older woman – the excess body fat takes raw materials and converts them into estrogen, and IGF-1 levels will increase too."

A number of scientists who research diet-hormone interactions are of the mind that obesity is a key factor in causing hormone-related cancers. One of these is Dr. Jin-Rong (Joseph) Zhou, Assistant Professor of Surgery at Harvard's Beth Israel Deaconess Medical Center. "Obesity and insulin resistance affect hormone levels, and these may be the bridge between dietary risk factors and the greater risk for hormone-related cancers," Dr. Zhou told me. "Obesity increases levels of the enzyme *aromatase*. This converts testosterone to estrogen in women, which raises breast cancer risk." Losing excess weight can obviously benefit women, but men can also benefit from the same, because the enzyme (5-alpha-reductase) that converts testosterone to its more dangerous [prostate-cancer-growing] form (dihydrotestosterone, DHT) is reduced by over 20% when men slim down.

So if the aim is to lower levels of hormones that would otherwise raise cancer risk, losing excess weight is clearly a main goal. However, weight loss is hard, and for many people it can be *very* difficult, even more so when preventing weight regain is thrown into the mix. Are there other ways to accomplish this goal without losing a large amount of weight?

The answer is, yes, yes, and yes – there are three other ways to achieve lower hormone levels that are definitely less challenging. These include reducing your fat intake, increasing your fiber, and getting some aerobic exercise.

Reducing fat intake lowers hormone levels

Evidence that fat intake influences blood hormones began to be uncovered roughly two decades ago, when Australian researchers compared hormone levels in women in response to either of two diets. One of these contained 40% of calories from fat, the other 20%. The Aussie team found that the lower fat diet not only reduced both estrogen and testosterone in women, but specifically lowered estradiol (the form of estrogen more often linked to breast cancer) more than other types of estrogen. Other investigators found that a low fat diet cuts down on production of the hormone *prolactin*. High prolactin levels are also related to two common diseases women experience that are strong risk factors for breast cancer (fibrocystic breast disease and cyclic mastalgia, or breast pain). After 3 months on a low fat (20% of calories) diet, previously elevated prolactin levels normalized. However, fat isn't the only nutrient that raises prolactin; high protein meals also increase this hormone, while high-carbohydrate meals don't seem to do so.

In terms of an actual payoff of eating less fat, data are mixed on breast cancer risk. It's difficult to separate the effects of eating less fat from the effect of losing weight from low fat dieting. In the Women's Intervention Nutrition Study (WINS), those who followed a lower fat diet experienced a decrease in breast cancer recurrence. Dr. Cheryl Rock commented on this study when we spoke of her research on fat, fiber, hormones and breast cancer.

"This study was done with a select group of women," she began. "They had to start out eating more than 35% of calories from fat, and be both post-menopausal and diagnosed with breast cancer. Would this strategy work as well for *pre*menopausal women or for ones *already* eating lower-fat diets? We just don't know." Surely enough, the Women's Healthy Eating and Living (WHEL) study published by Dr. Rock and her co-workers after we spoke showed no significant reduction in breast cancer recurrence or survival in women eating a lower-fat diet *and* more fiber, fruit, and vegetables. Although these two studies appear to contradict each other, an important difference between these two groups of women was bodyweight. Those in the WINS study weighed roughly 6 lbs. less on average than the WHEL study women as a result of their efforts to cut fat. Weighing more and eating more fat appears to increase the recurrence of breast cancer and shorten survival time.

Other studies have also suggested that *total* fat intake doesn't contribute to breast cancer, but that specific *types* of fats do. Saturated fats in red meat, dairy products, and egg yolk have been blamed, for a number of reasons. On the other hand, much evidence indicates that using olive oil as the main fat in your diet can lower your cancer risk, and the (omega-3) fat in fish may also be helpful. Higher fish intake is inversely related to the risk for colorectal cancer, and eating more fish has been linked to a much lower risk for *advanced* prostate cancers (not total incidence of this cancer).

The protein problem: how America's favorite nutrient raises your cancer risk

You probably haven't noticed it, but Americans are totally protein-obsessed. We've been programmed by the food industry, and to a certain degree by the nutrition community, to think of protein as something that we can't get too much of. As a result, thousands of food labels proudly proclaim their protein content, even when they are foods that people buy mainly for their value as a source of carbohydrates (breakfast cereal and granola bars, for example.)

The result, as government studies have shown, is that the U.S. is the highest consumer of meat out of all the developed nations. Adult women eat one and one-half times the amount they need, while men eat twice as much. This should come as no surprise, because most people plan their meals around their protein foods, although we only need less of it than carbs or fats. There are several problems related to our protein excess, including raising your cancer risk. How does animal protein do this?

First of all, overeating in *any* way will make you gain weight. This will go double if your protein sources are loaded with fat (as many are). Many sources of protein in our diets are also high in animal fat, the kind that contains most saturated fat and cholesterol. These include red meat, eggs, cheese, and whole milk. Cancer cells need this cholesterol at a certain stage in their development, and robbing them of it has the same growth-depriving effect as taking milk from a baby. If the cholesterol remains available, the inflammation it causes literally feeds the cancer machine over a long period of time, resulting in a tumor's increased ability to make more cancer cells (proliferation).

Another problem with high protein diets is that they increase hormone exposure through lowering sex hormone binding globulins (SHBG). Replacing animal protein with plant protein (for instance, soy products and other legumes, nuts and seeds, and meat substitutes) can reverse this step. This change explains to some degree why vegans and vegetarians enjoy a lower risk for some cancers.

Animal protein is also a major source of a certain kind of fat that drives cancer growth. Basically, there are three main types of fats, designated by the word 'omega' with a number next to it. The omega-3 fatty acids include a (short chain) fat found in canola oil, walnuts, flax seed, soybean oil, and green vegetables, and two ('long chain') types found in fish (EPA and DHA); olive oil is mostly an omega-9 fat. The type you should be most concerned about if you want to keep your cancer chances low is an omega-6 fat found in animal products called *arachidonic acid* (AA for short). Cancer cells take this fat and run it through two pathways (CO and LO).

What comes out are a number of hormone-like products that promote cancer cell growth and survival, angiogenesis, and metastasis, along with changes in your immune system (decreased immunity with increased inflammation) that heavily favor your chances of getting a cancer.

Eating more fiber lowers hormone levels

As we age and our minds slow down, digestion does too. The recommendations we receive from friends may change from what the hottest new music groups are to which kind of bran cereal works best. However, there are other reasons why you should adopt a higher fiber intake long before you get any older. In terms of reducing your risk for common, hormone-related cancers, eating more fiber-containing foods may be just what you're missing out on.

According to Dr. Rock, higher fiber intake is linked with a healthier hormone profile that is less likely to cause cancer. "Eating a high fiber diet was found in studies both in animals and humans to interfere with the normal cycle of estrogen," explained Dr. Rock. "Most people don't know this, but estrogen normally comes out in bile, goes into the gut, and is re-absorbed into the blood. A high fiber diet binds some of that estrogen, like it would cholesterol, and it winds up being excreted – resulting in decreased levels of estrogen in the blood." Dr. Rock continued by describing why fiber may be more important for controlling hormones than other nutrients are. "We found that in women who ate the most fiber, more vegetables and fruits, and less fat, that there was in fact a lowering of blood estrogen levels. When we tried to 'tease out' which dietary factors were most responsible for the effect, we found that fiber was actually more important than fat," she concluded.

Not surprisingly, high fiber, low fat diets affect male hormones too. When compared to a typical Western diet, the lower fat/high fiber meals reduce testosterone levels. However, this change alone may not impact prostate cancer risk, because testosterone itself isn't the problem. Instead, the target for prostate cancer prevention and treatment is the breakdown product of this hormone (dihydrotestosterone, DHT) and the enzyme that triggers the testosterone-to-DHT conversion. But if such a diet results in weight loss, so much the better: men who lose excess weight have lower levels of insulin and of the enzyme (5-alpha-reductase) that converts testosterone to DHT. Both these changes may help to lower the risk for prostate cancer.

Hormones with anti-cancer effects: the gift of melatonin

Melatonin, a hormone that is responsible to a great degree for how well we sleep, is one of the 'good' hormones that may lower the risk for hormone-related cancers. However, a shift from the sun-based lighting system we lived in centuries ago, in which light was limited to roughly 12 hours each day, to an electricity-based system, providing light for several additional hours, has subtracted from this natural anti-cancer mechanism. This excess light suppresses your melatonin production, and you start to lose the anti-cancer benefits that come with it. These include antioxidant, anti-estrogen, and anti-angiogenesis effects, control of abnormal cell division, and the ability to trigger apoptosis and differentiation (discussed below) and boost immunity.

These conclusions have been long in coming. However, solid evidence has shown that situations related to light exposure, including population level community nighttime light levels (for example, living in cities) and night shift work, increase cancer risk. On the other hand, situations in which light exposure is non-existent (blindness, for example) or limited (long sleep duration) lower cancer risk. Light exposure is the main, but not the only influence on melatonin; being older, overweight, and smoking are all related to lower melatonin output, and even diet plays a role.

When connections between melatonin and cancer were first established, it was due to the finding of an increased risk for breast cancer in night shift nurses. Breast cancer risk is, as research has recently revealed, only the tip of the iceberg as far as melatonin deficiency and cancer goes. Working night shifts also increase the risk for endometrial, colorectal, and prostate cancers, as well as non-Hodgkin's lymphoma.

Can increasing melatonin lower cancer risk? The data don't yet indicate this, but it is convincing with respect to cancer *treatment*. Two recent publications from separate groups of scientists looked at all available studies that used melatonin supplements alone or in combination with chemotherapy and radiation. Both research groups concluded that high doses of melatonin substantially improved chances for remission from cancer, survival at 1 year after treatment, and alleviated the side effects of radiation and chemotherapy.

At this point, you might be wondering why I'm writing about a hormone like melatonin, and its use as a supplement, in a book about food and cancer. As it turns out, melatonin is both a hormone *and* a phytochemical – it's found in walnuts, bananas, grain products, and vegetables. Interestingly, women who eat the most vegetables excrete 16% more melatonin breakdown products in their urine than those with the lowest vegetable intake. This may turn out to be important for reducing breast cancer risk, given that that women with higher urinary melatonin output were found to have a nearly a 45% lower risk for invasive breast cancer. It's not unreasonable to suspect that melatonin in foods complements the anti-cancer effects of the phytochemicals, vitamins, minerals, and fiber in a healthy diet.

Vitamin D

Unless you've studied nutrition or had other schooling in the health field, you're probably not aware that vitamin D does double-duty as a vitamin and a hormone. Although it takes a few steps to convert the former to the latter, the results are critical for cancer prevention. And consider this while you're reading: vitamin D deficiency is considered to be epidemic in the U.S. How bad *is* this situation? It varies, as most research efforts do, from one study to another. However, one group of physicians conducting a chart review of patients in their general practice found that 87% were mildly to severely deficient. A study on patients attending a rehab clinic found that 67% were either insufficient or deficient. Experts in this area have chimed in with numbers close to these, estimating that a full 75% of adults have low vitamin D levels. Keep this figure in mind as you read what's coming up on the relationship between this hormone and cancer risk.

The hormone form of vitamin D affects several critically important cancer growth stages, including angiogenesis; cancer proliferation (the creation of more cells); apoptosis; and differentiation. Being more specific, let's take the examples of two of the most common cancers. Blood levels of one form of vitamin D are inversely related (meaning, higher levels mean lower risk, and vice versa) not only with breast cancer development, but also risk for breast cancer recurrence and risk for dying. The same inverse relationship has been found for vitamin D and your risk for colorectal cancer. Breast cancer is the most common cancer in women, affecting 1 out of 8, and colorectal cancer, the third most common cancer, affects 1 out of 20 persons here in the U.S. In other words, unless you're getting a fair amount of sun each week or taking a vitamin D supplement, you could be at risk for one, or even both, of these cancers.

A final reason it's important to rein in your hormones is that they increase the ability of cancer cells to duplicate themselves, a process known as proliferation. I'll provide some details of this below, along with several ways phytochemical-containing foods helps to restrain this process.

Cell cycles: Wheels of misfortune

Given that there are literally hundreds of types of cancer, it's impressive that they all share one characteristic: disruption of normal controls that keep their growth in check. When researchers talk about this process, they use the word *proliferation*, a term made up in part of two smaller words: 'pro' and 'life'. In order for cells to proliferate, they need to go through a 'cell cycle' consisting of the several phases that (if you remember your high school biology) constitute mitosis: a resting ('Gap', or G0) phase, a DNA synthesis ('S') phase, a second 'Gap' phase (G1), and a mitosis ('M') phase.

Progression from one part of the cell cycle to another is a result in part of an excess of growth factors (IGF-1, insulin, and epidermal growth factor, EGF) and certain hormones. These can trigger cancer proliferation through the action of proteins called *cyclins* and *cyclin-dependent kinases* (CDKs). The several kinds of cyclins are expressed as letters (A, B, and so forth). For example, cyclin D1 controls the transition from the G1 (resting) to the critical DNA synthesis ('S') phase. "Cyclins are catalysts in this process, ones that are over-expressed in most cancers," explained Dr. Raj Agarwal, a University of Colorado Professor who has studied the effects of phytochemicals on the cell cycle.

Phytochemicals also impact other controls on cell proliferation, including *Activator protein* 1 (AP-1), mutations in certain genes (*ras, raf*), *tyrosine kinases*, and oxidative stress. In later chapters, I'll discuss how specific phytochemicals in whole grains, green tea, soy foods, and fruits and vegetables have the ability to interfere with the functioning of cyclins and CDKs, which is a key to how these foods help lower cancer risk.

How growth factors turn the wheel on the cell cycle

Growth factors, if you remember, are proteins that both inhibit apoptosis and increase the risk for cancer metastasis by enabling angiogenesis. They also push the cell cycle forward. When epidermal growth factor (EGF), IGF-1 or other growth factors combine with receptors on a cell's surface, the result is the sending of a message to the cell's nucleus for a cell to divide. This message-sending process from the cell surface to the inside of the cell, known as 'signal transduction,' is carried or amplified by the ras gene and by proteins ('kinases'), in what's been likened to a 'bucket brigade' of cancer growth signals.

Dr. Agarwal has published extensively on this topic, and during our conversation he noted that growth factors and their receptors both have critical roles in the cancer cell cycle. "When growth factors and their receptors interact, they produce a growth signal," he began. "That signal tells the cells to divide. This happens under normal conditions too, but cancer cells actually make more receptors. The most important growth factors are EGF and its receptors," he continued. The proof of the importance of growth factors like EGF, he noted, is indicated by development and use of the drug Herceptin® (Trastuzumab), an antibody that prevents cancer proliferation by targeting an EGF-related protein that's critical to the growth of certain breast cancers.

Several foods may affect the amount of EGF humans are exposed to, including red meat, soy foods, broccoli, and green tea. One interesting study found links between diet, different forms of the EGF gene ('polymorphisms'), and breast cancer risk in younger women. Along with finding individual differences in the EGF gene, a diet analysis of those who ate the most red meat (> 65 grams per day, slightly over 2 ounces) *and* had a strong family history of breast cancer exposed some fascinating links between diet, genes, and cancer risk. Frequent red meat eaters with certain EGF polymorphisms had roughly 11 times greater a risk for breast cancer compared with those who ate the least red meat. By comparison, women with the high-risk EGF genes who ate the most vegetables (about 12.5 ounces) had the *lowest* cancer risk.

EGF is also found in foods. One commonly consumed source (probably the *main* source) is cow's milk and milk products. EGF is *supposed* to be in milk – it's a growth factor, meant to grow babies and calves. We don't yet know a lot of things about possible risks from EGF in cow's milk, including whether or not humans absorb EGF from dairy foods, or if the EGF in dairy products would increase cancer risk even if we did absorb it. However, we can't say that there's absolutely no cause for concern, because some studies have concluded that drinking milk has been associated with a higher risk for cancers of the lung, pancreas, prostate, ovaries, endometrium, and for lymphoma. These findings have to be considered with the strong evidence of an inverse association between milk intake and risk of colorectal and bladder cancers. Until this has been sorted out, I would recommend that you use soy milk and soy cheese in place of dairy. The isoflavones found in soy foods actually block the EGF receptor, and soy has cholesterol-lowering benefits that dairy products don't have. When you do consume dairy products, consider getting them from a source that contains probiotics, such as kefir or a probiotic-fortified yogurt. These can simultaneously boost your immunity while reducing inflammation, both of which may lower your cancer risk.

Activator protein-1: the spokes on the wheel

Activator protein 1 (AP-1) is a 'transcription' factor, which is science-speak for making a record, a copy. With respect to cancer, AP-1's role is to increase the production of cyclins that are involved in cell division, such as cyclin D1, an excess of which is linked to cancers of the breast, head and neck, lung, oral cavity, and cervix.

Certain stressors can increase AP-1. One of these is drinking too much alcohol; another is high blood sugar, which helps to explain why people with diabetes get cancer more often. However, It may not even be necessary for you to have diabetes to experience this risk. A study in humans found that a large rise in blood sugar after drinking 300 sugar calories (about as much as you'd get from a 16 ounce soda or fruit drink) increases AP-1. Oxidative stress, which happens when we smoke, are chronically ill, or make it a habit to eat diets low in antioxidants and high in saturated fat and refined carbs, also raises AP-1.

Under experimental conditions, a large number of antioxidant phytochemicals in foods have revealed the ability to decrease AP-1, including resveratrol, curcumin (found in turmeric and curry powder), gingerol (a phytochemical found in ginger), capsaicin (found in red pepper) catechins (found in tea and many fruits and vegetables), nobiletin (found in tangerines), cranberry, apple peel extract, lycopene, and a class of phytochemicals (isothiocyanates) found in the cruciferous vegetables, including broccoli, cabbage, and cauliflower. Phytochemicals in green tea (EGCG, ECG, theaflavin) also inhibit both AP-1 *and* EGF. These have worked under experimental conditions only so far. However, there's reason to believe they work in the human body also. One study that compared a low-antioxidant olive oil with antioxidant-rich oil (similar to the difference between a refined olive oil and the extra virgin type) and found that the higher quality oil reduced AP-1 and other mediators of cancer risk. These effects explain, to some degree, the relationships seen between olive oil use, Mediterranean diets, and lower cancer risk.

Putting the brakes on the cell cycle

Tumor suppressor genes are critical for slowing down or stopping cell division and causing cell cycle arrest. The 'p53' gene, one of the best known tumor suppressor genes (although the breast cancer gene *BRCA* has probably gotten more press) creates a protein that allows cells to recognize if any damage has occurred, and to trigger a 'fix it or nix it' response to that damage. While the repair crews are at work, p53 puts a hold on cell cycle progression. As the most commonly affected gene in human cancer, p53 mutations occur in more than 50% of all tumors. P53 mutations have been related to diet, and linked with higher intakes of both red meat and total meat, and between 3% and10% of these are estimated to be the result of eating the chemical by-products of cooking meats.

Dr. Martha Slattery, a Professor of Epidemiology at the University of Utah, has published several studies on how diet may affect p53 mutations. She explained the roles of tumor suppressor genes during a conversation we had about her research on patients with colon cancer. "Tumor suppressor genes regulate cell growth," she began. "P53 and another tumor suppressor gene called the retinoblastoma (Rb) gene are mutated in many cancers, making them non-functional." Dr. Slattery and her co-workers found that 40%-50% of patients in their study had p53 mutations. In addition, they detailed possible interactions between diet and gene mutations that could trigger cancer proliferation. "We observed some specific associations between p53 mutations and factors present in a Western-style diet," Dr. Slattery continued. "We think these observations support other studies showing relationships between diet and colon cancer." Specifically, Dr. Slattery and her co-workers found that persons with p53 mutations were twice as likely to be eating a Western diet (animal products, white flour and sugar, and low in fruits, vegetables, and whole grains) as those without mutations. Most of the risk appeared due to red meat, fast food, and *trans* fats, the type found in partially hydrogenated vegetable oils used in fast food and processed foods. They also found that patients eating more processed meats, such as bacon, hot dogs, and sausage, were more likely to have mutations in *ras* (a gene controlling cancer proliferation). Italian researchers came to similar conclusions, finding p53 mutations more common among consumers of diets higher in milk, meat, sugars, animal fat, and nitrite.

In contrast to these other foods, carbohydrates may offer some protection from this process, if we eat the right ones. Studies in human volunteers found that eating more fruits and vegetables were protective against p53 mutation. On the other hand, Dr. Slattery and her co-workers found evidence that eating *refined* carbohydrates with a high glycemic index (those that raise blood sugar very quickly) might contribute to cancer risk. In one of these studies, women eating a diet high in these foods were at greater risk for p53 mutations. In a later study, women who had a combination of high sugar intake and greater estrogen exposure had roughly three times the risk for a p53 mutation. Dr. Slattery and her co-workers also found *ras* mutations more often in patients eating high-fat diets and refined carbs. "We actually observed that a high glycemic index [diet] in women can increase p53 mutations," Dr. Slattery summarized. "We're not sure how this happens, but we think it may be regulated by estrogen and inflammation-related pathways."

Antioxidants to the rescue

Keeping cancer cells from proliferating is an important goal of cancer prevention and treatment, and inhibiting cyclins gets this done. In turn, this is accomplished by the cyclin-dependent kinase inhibitors (CDKIs), which are designated with a 'p' – p15, p15, p21, p27 and so forth.

Getting more phytochemicals in your diet can do a number of important things to stop the cancer cell cycle. Dr. Agarwal pointed out that these foods contribute to an antioxidant effect, which helps inhibit a master regulator of the body's inflammatory response (nuclear factor kappa B, NFκB). Restraining NFκB decreases cyclin D1, the most important of the cyclins. Antioxidant phytochemicals also prevent the *ras* gene from causing cell cycle progression. "The first thing phytochemicals can do is inhibit growth signals," Dr. Agarwal explained. "If they do so, CDKs will not be activated. The second thing is they can induce CDK inhibitor proteins (CDKIs); third, they inhibit the *breakdown* of CDKIs. Fourth, they can decrease the level of cyclins."

Several foods and beverages contain phytochemicals that have the ability to interfere with cyclins and CDKs. These include inositol hexaphosphate (found in whole grains and legumes); green tea; carotenoids found in tomatoes; soy foods; cruciferous vegetables; and *quercetin*, a phytochemical found in a wide range of fruits and vegetables (including apples, onions, tomatoes, grapes and berries, and buckwheat). Eating more of these can help to interfere with cancer proliferation, but they may not be enough to inhibit cancer growth unless accompanied by other, more stringent changes in diet. I found this out by questioning Dr. Fazlul Sarkar, a Professor of Pathology (and an incredibly prolific cancer researcher) at Wayne State University in Detroit. I interviewed Dr. Sarkar regarding his work on soy and cancer prevention, and asked him if the average person could attain a lower cancer risk simply by adding some phytochemical-rich foods to an otherwise poor or Western diet. "If you have a high level of IGF signaling going, then many of these otherwise protective phytochemicals are going to be ineffective for stopping the cell cycle," he began. "To be more specific, if you have a lot of meat products and such in your diet, no matter how many fruits and vegetables you eat, it won't be beneficial. *It's like putting one foot on the accelerator and one foot on the brake, and you won't be able to stop cancer cell growth"* [italics mine].

Having an abundance of meat (and other animal) products in your diet also affects your immune system in ways that dangerously impact cancer growth. I'll explain some of the ways this happens below, and will (in a later chapter) give you specific examples of how phytochemical-containing foods can 'tune' your immune system to both kill cancers and restrain inflammation.

Immunity, Inflammation, Diet and Cancer

Out of a number of roadblocks to cancer development the body presents, your immune system represents the last. In this section, I'll describe how your immune system can prevent cancer growth or encourage it, beginning with an explanation of how immunity works as an 'eye in the sky' that watches over cancer development. With some help from scientists I spoke with, I'll also explain some general ways in which your immunity impacts your cancer risk through nutritional deficits, excesses, and through inflammation.

Immunosurveillance and cancer prevention

The study of the impact of the immune system on cancer can be traced back almost a full century to Paul Ehrlich, a German bacteriologist, who was the first scientist to suggest that the immune system might act in a surveillance mode against malignancy. Suspicion increased when clinicians working with patients who were either immune-suppressed or who were given medications to suppress immunity (after organ transplantation) observed an increase in cancers in these patients. When HIV (in which critical T-cells are lacking) started affecting greater numbers of persons in the 1980's, cancers caused by poor immunity (e.g., Kaposi's sarcoma) were increasingly seen. Interestingly, even without HIV, persons with less aggressive T-cells are at greater cancer risk, and the reverse is also true: cancer risk is lower in persons with *more* aggressive T-cells.

Since then, scientists have published evidence indicating that your immune system's T-cells and B-cells destroy the vast majority of malignant cells before they can manifest as cancer. Immune activity may also be responsible for 'tumor dormancy,' a state in which cancers may be kept clinically silent, asleep and not growing for months and even years. In fact, immune surveillance-related tumor dormancy has been estimated in breast cancer patients to last *up to 25 years*. Conceivably then, keeping your immune system in good condition could make the difference between being told you have a cancer at age 60 and being diagnosed at 85 years of age – a possible difference of roughly one-third of a normal life span for many people.

How is this possible? One pathway may be through your immune system's ability to suppressing the growth of certain viruses, which are thought to be responsible for roughly 15%

of human cancers. The human papilloma virus (HPV), which causes cervical cancer and is present in 3 out of every 4 adults in the U.S., is a perfect example. HPV can now (thankfully) by vaccinated against. However, many Nutritionists find it very interesting that several studies have indicated a relationship may exist between nutrition, immunity, and growth of HPV. Specifically, researchers found the strongest evidence for protection against HPV-induced cancer in women who got more vitamin A, vitamin E and folate in their diets. Expert review of the data on this topic called the evidence 'possible' that higher intakes of fruits and vegetables, vitamins C and B12, and carotenoids (alpha- and beta carotene, lycopene, lutein/zeaxanthin and cryptoxanthin) also helped to get rid of the HPV infection. These benefits were suggested to be due to an ability of these nutrients to enhance immune function and decrease viral replication.

There's also evidence that other phytochemicals (flavonoids) might protect you against virus-induced cancers. Scientists have known for roughly forty years that many flavonoids have anti-viral effects. More recently, flavonoids were found to inhibit the growth of human rhinoviruses (the kind that cause the common cold). These effects had previously been seen only under experimental conditions. However, Korean scientists found that green tea extracts also inhibited growth of HPV in women with cervical lesions (warts), whether it was applied as an ointment or taken in pill form. Japanese scientists studying the antiviral effects of flavonoids in green tea found that these could inhibit the growth of leukemia cells and the virus that causes leukemia (human T-cell lymphotropic virus, HTLV-1), and decided to perform a clinical trial with green tea in virus-infected human subjects. Their study, which involved giving HTLV-1-infected men a green tea extract in capsule form, found that taking the extract for 5 months resulted in a significantly lower amount of virus in their blood, compared to men not getting the tea extract. Successfully treating leukemia with green tea is also a strong possibility; the Mayo Clinic's hematology division documented that 3 of 4 patients taking green tea supplements obtained partial responses to another form of leukemia (chronic lymphocytic leukemia, CLL). CLL is a cancer that is characterized by a failure of immune cells to undergo apoptosis, which happens to be one of the ways that green tea reduces cancer risk. This combination of both viral inhibition and apoptosis induction make green tea a powerful potential anti-cancer strategy for leukemia, as well as many other cancers.

In people who are already fighting cancer, reduced immune function may also be responsible for cancer progression. On the other hand, some evidence indicates that getting more immune-boosting nutrients may improve prognosis. One way better nutrition may impact cancer survival is through an effect on a specific type of immune cell called a 'natural killer' cell, the most important type in cancer prevention.

Natural killer (NK) cells get their well-deserved name comes from the evidence that it's in their nature to destroy suspected invaders before they strike first. Unlike other immune cells that work by launching chemical weapons or recruiting other immune cells, the uniqueness of natural killer cells comes from two important abilities. First, natural killer cells play important roles in immunosurveillance. NK cells have an ability to kill malignant cells on the spot, without being prompted or recruited like other immune cells. Even better, they *selectively* kill malignant cells, and are thought to help prevent metastasis. This last trait may explain why poor natural killer cell function is tied to a worse prognosis in cancer patients and an increased risk for cancer recurrence after cancer surgery. Natural killer cells also help to induce other kinds of immune cells (T-cells) and chemical weapons they produce (cytokines) that defend against cancer.

Your NK cells, like all the other cells you possess, respond to changes in your diet, for better or worse. For instance, they may not function well without enough zinc or selenium, but cutting down fat intake has been shown to improve NK cell function.

Fat intake, immunity, and cancer risk

Of all the nutrients that impact your immunity, inflammation, and cancer risk, dietary fat is probably the most critical. And out of all the types of fat in our diet, an excess of saturated fat and cholesterol from red meat, high-fat dairy products, and eggs may be the most significant cause of inflammation. In turn, inflammation is linked to cancer risk. I asked Dr. Darshan Kelley, a research chemist with the USDA's Western Human Nutrition Research Center (WHNRC), to give me some background on the role of fat in immune function and cancer.

Dr. Kelley has been researching and publishing articles on fat and immunity for over 20 years. He's also led the WHNRC's Project on Dietary Fat and Health since 1990. Specifically, his work has focused on the effects on immunity of the amount and types of fat people eat.

"A high fat intake *does* suppress immune function, and we've done studies showing that reducing fat improves immunity," he began. "Generally, immunity improves when we bring fat intake down from 40% of calories to 35% of calories and then to 30%. So thirty percent of calories from fat is OK - it's more a question of the *type* of fat," he continued.

If you're trying to keep your cancer risk low, keep in mind that an omega-6 fat (arachidonic acid, AA), found in meat, poultry, eggs and fish is also undesirable. Most people know that omega-3 fats are good for our health; what they *don't* know is that AA is the 'evil twin' of these two classes of fats. These two exist in a 'Jekyll and Hyde' kind of relationship, and when there are not enough omega-3's and inflammation occurs, our bodies use AA to make hormone-like chemicals that influence immunity, inflammation, and cancer growth. The most important of these, prostaglandin E2 (PGE2), suppresses immunity, including that of natural killer cells. At the same time, PGE2 also increases inflammation, drives cell division, and results in faster tumor growth. "PGE2 and another fat-derived chemical called LTB4 increase as we raise the amount of omega-6 fats in our diets," Dr. Kelley explained. "Both the linoleic acid in vegetable oils and the arachidonic acid (AA) found in animal products create these, but the arachidonic acid is far more potent." (To give you an idea of how important these hormone-like chemicals are for cancer growth, consider that blocking their production with aspirin, ibuprofen and similar products is thought to help prevent cancers of the breast, lung, stomach, colon, rectum, and esophagus, and possibly prostate cancer).

Most people should strictly limit the intake of animal products because of the saturated fat and cholesterol they contain, due to the risk for cardiovascular disease. However, there are two other reasons for doing so that figure in to your cancer risk. The first is the presence of a carbohydrate named *Neu5Gc* found in red meat and dairy products. Neu5Gc accumulates in human tumors, causing your immune cells to invade tumors and enhance both their growth and angiogenesis. In addition, red meat, high-fat dairy products (butter and cream cheese, for example) and broiled, fried, grilled, and roasted meats contain 'advanced glycation end products', or *glycotoxins*, that add to your cancer risk through inflammation. Glycotoxins accumulate to a greater degree in persons with diabetes, and represent one reason why this disease increases cancer risk above that of people without this disease.

As to why a chronic low-level inflammation increases cancer risk, there are several mechanisms. These include favoring angiogenesis, decreasing apoptosis, and damaging your DNA. The link between inflammation and cancer is evident in persons who are unlucky enough to have chronic inflammatory diseases. These include inflammatory bowel diseases (ulcerative colitis and Crohn's disease) as well as hepatitis, *H pylori* infection (found in 29%-60% of U.S. residents), chronic lung disease, and certain other diseases where your immune system gets stuck in high gear. The risk of cancer due to inflammation appears to be the result of a vicious cycle in which immune cells produce free radicals, *cytokines*, and *chemokines* that further amplify the immune response. This response then produces more free radicals that can damage DNA or interfere with DNA repair. Inflammation can also release growth factors and cytokines that promote cancer growth.

Phytochemicals, inflammation and cancer

Rather than stimulating immunity like many vitamins and minerals do, most phytochemicals work the opposite end of the immune equation by suppressing excess inflammation. One of the ways they do so is similar to how aspirin and other such drugs (NSAID's, non-steroidal anti-inflammatory drugs) work. But here's the catch: these phytochemicals are spread out among different classes of edibles. Some are in whole grains, fruits and vegetables; some in beverages like tea, hot chocolate and coffee; and others are found in herbs and spices, including curry powder, garlic, and ginger, among many others. A truly anti-inflammatory diet is plant-based; it doesn't necessarily exclude animal products. Rather, it maximizes plant foods, beverages and spices, while using animal products in small amounts to complement the meal, not *as* the meal.

Exercise, lifestyle choices and inflammation

Moderate exercise does a marvelous job of balancing immunity and inflammation that nicely complements what smart eating will do. Exercisers also get colds less often, a benefit that might be due to having a higher white blood cell count or greater oral secretion of salivary immunoglobulin A (sIgA), an antibody that forms our first line of defense against infection. At the same time, moderate regular exercise suppresses inflammation both short- and long-term. Keep it moderate, though: excessive, exhaustive exercise can have the opposite effect you'd want, by suppressing immunity while increasing inflammation.

As you might guess, smoking is not an option if turning off inflammation is your goal. Alcohol is another story, however. As with most things, moderation is a key to a balanced immune system. Alcohol's effects are dependent on the dose; moderate use is associated with a reduction of inflammation, while heavy drinking increases inflammation.

What the immune system damages, the body must repair, if we're to remain intact. Unfortunately, we don't get to *stay* intact; DNA damage builds up throughout our lives, and is a fundamental, critical means by which people age and develop cancers. There are two ways that you can help your body deal with this damage. The first is by protecting your DNA from being damaged in the first place. The second way is to make sure you have what your DNA needs for its repair mechanisms to work up to par.

Healthy DNA: Diet, DNA damage & DNA repair

As I discussed in the section on toxins and detoxification, one of the anti-cancer benefits of eating a diet higher in plant foods and less animal foods is that we take in less (and excrete more) DNA-damaging toxins. DNA damage is an underlying cause of mutations leading to cancer, and people who have a poorer ability to repair DNA damage are at greater cancer risk. Humans have evolved 4 ways to handle this type of damage: apoptosis; control of cell cycle checkpoints; damage tolerance, and DNA repair. Of all these, DNA repair is the most effective, because it directly removes lesions from DNA. In spite of its relevance to cancer prevention, studying DNA repair has been the focus of very few scientists. "It's clear that DNA repair is crucially important," commented Dr. Andrew Collins, a Professor in Nutrition at Norway's University of Oslo. "But there's not much work being done on the effect of nutrition on this process, although a lot of attention has been paid to the role of antioxidants in preventing DNA damage. The field of diet-related DNA repair is under-funded, and it's quite frustrating."

Causes and measurement of DNA damage

If you want to know whether or not your DNA is taking hits, look first to your lifestyle habits. These preventable causes of DNA damage, which include smoking, poor diet, and excessive drinking, will be important influences on your production of DNA-damaging free radicals. If you're a smoker, you should expect a 150% greater amount of DNA damage compared to non-smokers. The people around you will be at a similar disadvantage, because second-hand smoke also inflicts damage on DNA. Working with chemicals, exposure to ultraviolet light and other forms of radiation, and drugs (legal or illegal) can also damage your DNA. If you're concerned about cancer risk, you can often choose to leave these avoidable causes of DNA damage behind.

Just as there are avoidable causes of DNA damage, there are unavoidable causes too. Gender is one, and guys are on the losing end. DNA damage to a crucial part of human cells (the mitochondria, the source of all our energy) is 4 times higher in males than in females. The decrease in DNA damage found in women compared with men is thought to be due in part to estrogen, and specifically to the fact that this hormone increases the amount of DNA-protecting antioxidant enzymes. Unfortunately, men don't have a greater rate of DNA repair than women to help us compensate. This may account for at least part of why, generally speaking, women have a lower mortality rate from cancer than men. However, exposure to toxins also results in greater DNA damage in newborns, thereby raising their future cancer risk. Although these types of results have been documented mainly in animal studies, an investigation by Columbia University researchers found the same results in humans. In a cross-sectional study of 67 mothers and 64 newborns from the Krakow Region of Poland, results showed a typical indicator of DNA damage (DNA adducts; defined as DNA bonded to a carcinogen that could be the start of a cancerous cell) were found in high amounts in the blood and umbilical cords of newborns exposed to air pollutants through the mother's placenta.

DNA damage is measured in a number of ways, but the one most commonly used by scientists is the level of 8-OHdG in urine. There are however, some problems with this marker, and Dr. Cynthia Thompson, a registered dietitian and researcher at the Arizona Cancer Center, provided some explanation. "8-OHdG is the most reputable marker, but the problem with 8-OHdG is that it's highly variable in a person from day to day," she began. "So if we measure your 8-OHdG levels on three consecutive days, there's a good chance we're going to see up to 40% variation. Investigators have addressed this by collecting samples on several consecutive days and using pooled [averaged] samples to estimate 8-OHdG, before and after diet interventions," she added. There is also some disagreement over what 8OHdG measures, as Dr. Thompson explained. "The current thinking is that if OH-8dG levels go down, that's a sign of improvement in health status. This is somewhat controversial, because some think that putting out less 8-OHdG means that a person is less able to do repair." Nevertheless, several studies show a higher amount of 8OHdG in people who are exposed to toxins, or who later develop cancer, or who have cancer, compared to healthy persons. And, as I'll discuss in detail below, people who eat healthier often have lower levels of 8OHdG than those who eat poorly.

How your diet affects DNA damage

Other than smoking or the daily ingestion of other toxins, your food intake will probably be your greatest preventable source of DNA damage. Specifically, the balance between antioxidants and pro-oxidants in your diet will affect this. Accordingly, manufacturers of teas and fruit juices have worked hard to advertise their products as antioxidant-rich. The widespread availability of healthy foods and beverages in the United States has also made antioxidants fairly easy to find in or food supply, *if* you care to search for these. On the other side of the coin, most foods found in grocery stores and fast food restaurants are worthless, as far as DNA health (and health in general) is concerned. Food scientists proved this in an article published in the *American Journal of Clinical Nutrition* by analyzing a spectrum of typically eaten foods found in the Western diet. Meats, dairy products, white flour grain products, convenience foods and other staples of the American diet were studied to determine their antioxidant capacity. Practically none had *any* ability to neutralize free radical damage. The only exception, humorously enough, were certain snack foods, specifically, the *chocolate*-containing ones!

Unfortunately, DNA-damaging *pro*-oxidants are easier to get. One important source of pro-oxidants is *oxysterols*. These are cholesterol oxidation products found mainly in eggs, but also in certain milk products and fried meats. Oxysterols are also made in your own body from LDL cholesterol, which gets oxidized fairly easily when we don't eat enough antioxidants. Interestingly, your body's response to oxidized LDL is to send an antibody to get rid of it. This sounds like a rescue mission, but it turns out to be a case of friendly fire, as it actually results in more DNA damage *and* a decrease in DNA repair enzyme activity.

Oxysterols sit side-by-side in foods with arachidonic acid (which, if you remember, is involved simultaneously in suppressing immunity and increasing inflammation). When Dr. Thompson and her colleagues asked 202 women with a history of breast cancer to record their food intake, they found that arachidonic acid intakes were associated with a greater degree of DNA damage. "A lot of publications have revealed an association between arachidonic acid and oxidative stress," Dr. Thompson confirmed. "This suggests there's a connection between inflammation, oxidative stress, and cancer."

More convincing evidence of a connection between diet and DNA damage was found by Italian investigators, who contrasted items in the food supplies of industrialized countries (Western nations, Asia, and parts of Europe) with the number of DNA mutations found in colon cancer. Although this study did not show cause and effect, it found significant correlations between the availability of meat, milk, sweeteners, animal fats, and DNA mutations.

If a diet that contains an abundance of animal foods, oxysterols, and AA increases DNA damage, can avoiding animal products decrease it? Some, but not all, studies seem to indicate this is so. Vegetarians appear to have a lower degree of DNA damage than meat-eaters. This may be due to getting more antioxidants and less pro-oxidants than omnivores, but whether or not antioxidants always protect against DNA damage is not exactly clear. It depends on which studies you read, how the study was conducted, how DNA damage was measured, the age, gender, and health status of subjects in the study, and other variables. Many studies have manipulated fruit and vegetable intakes to try and see if removing or adding these could change the degree of DNA damage. Dr. Collins described a study he and his team performed, in which adding three kiwifruits each day to the diets of healthy humans had significant DNA-protective effects. "We set out to detect if levels of vitamin C in the blood that were increased by eating kiwifruit translated into a decrease in DNA damage," he began. "When we took lymphocytes [white blood cells] out of the blood of people who'd been eating kiwifruit for a couple of weeks and compared these with persons not eating kiwi, we found a significantly lower amount of oxidative DNA damage." Other studies done in human volunteers at the University of Milan (Italy) found that DNA damage was reduced roughly 4% in humans drinking two cups of green tea each day, compared to those not drinking tea, and that drinking orange juice improved resistance against oxidative DNA damage by roughly 18%, although vitamin C alone didn't.

Surprisingly, a number of studies showed that foods you might think are DNA-protective had no relationship with DNA damage. One of these was an investigation by Dr. Peter Moller, a scientist with the University of Copenhagen's Institute of Public Health. Dr. Moller and I discussed work he and his colleagues published on diet and DNA damage, which were disappointing. In their study, they gave 43 healthy, non-smoking, normal weight men and women a diet free of fruits and vegetables, or one providing 5 servings per day. Knowing what we do about the ability of the antioxidants in fruits and vegetables to reduce free radicals, we would expect DNA damage to decrease. No such luck. The Copenhagen team found no evidence that a fruit and vegetable-enriched diet reduced DNA damage in the white blood cells of these volunteers. Neither was there an increase in DNA damage in subjects on diets free of fruits and vegetables. "We can tell people to eat more fruits and vegetables for other reasons, but we can't tell them for sure that it will protect their DNA against damage," commented Dr. Moller.

Other studies have also failed to reveal a protective effect on DNA of eating high-antioxidant foods or taking antioxidant supplements. In fact, only in roughly one-third of studies did food or antioxidant supplements reveal DNA-protective effects. The reason that benefits are not always found, Dr. Collins suggested, is that a benefit of antioxidants shows up mainly in individuals who have a greater amount of DNA damage to begin with: smokers, for instance, or people with poor diet and marginal antioxidant status. Dr. Thompson had another possible explanation. "Measurement error or dealing with an already healthy population where oxidative stress is already low and hard to further decrease could affect the results of the 8-OHdG test, which might explain why certain studies showed no benefit of diet intervention," she suggested.

There are actually better explanations than these, and the evidence comes from comparing two types of dietary *patterns*, rather than simply judging the impact of fruits or vegetables. Nutrition scientists know that our total antioxidant intake comes from a combination of whole grains, fruits and vegetables, legumes, beverages, and herbs and spices. To expect a change in DNA damage from one or two food groups (i.e., just increasing fruits and vegetables) may not be reasonable, especially if people are eating poor or Western diets. Evidence that dietary patterns are better predictors of DNA damage was found in studies that compared Mediterranean diets with a Western pattern in groups of healthy volunteers. Clear associations were found between higher intakes of phytochemicals and red wine, antioxidant capacity of the blood, and a lower amount of DNA damage on the Mediterranean diet. Dr. Collins summarized the conclusions of these studies, saying, "It may not be individual antioxidants that are protective against DNA damage; perhaps a mixture of the antioxidants presents in foods is responsible. It seems that a combination of antioxidants can work together to greater effect than when acting on their own. I suspect that even this is not the whole story. There are many other things phytochemicals could be doing, and one of them seems to be an enhancing effect on DNA repair."

Diet and DNA repair

DNA repair is fascinating for a number of reasons, but the one that stands out is that *DNA is the only large molecule that is repaired by your body, while everything else is merely replaced.* "DNA repair is sort of a 'second line' of defense within the body," Dr. Collins explained. "Once the damage to DNA has occurred in spite of the antioxidant defenses, almost all of it is repaired, and the quicker that's done the better."

Scientists have confirmed the cancer-preventive importance of DNA repair from two kinds of studies. One of these found that 'silencing' DNA repair genes accelerated the onset of cancer, aging and age-related diseases. The second came from the observation that people with a condition called *xeroderma pigmentosum* (a disease that increases susceptibility to skin cancer) have defective DNA repair. The importance of DNA repair became even clearer after the realization that differences in the efficiency of DNA repair genes we inherit ('polymorphisms') often affects the risk for specific cancers. Breast cancer, for instance, may be affected by a combination of defective DNA repair and two high-risk breast cancer genes, and the risk for certain forms of skin cancer may be similarly affected.

We can't change our inherited ability to repair our DNA, but we can maximize what we were given. The evidence is lean but accumulating, and it's starting to indicate that certain kinds of foods affect DNA stability. Antioxidant-rich diets should help, because they increase DNA repair *and* oppose the free radicals that impair DNA repair enzymes. Alcohol, a known carcinogen, produces free radicals and has a suppressive effect on some DNA repair enzymes, so moderation and high-antioxidant diets are indicated for drinkers. However, any diet that doesn't provide enough micronutrients may actually cause more harm than good by negatively affecting DNA integrity. So far, the list of nutrients we need for this purpose includes iron, zinc, vitamin C and D, several B-vitamins, and possibly calcium. According to Dr. Michael Fenech, the Project Leader of the Nutrigenomics and Genome Health Laboratory at Australia's Commonwealth Scientific and Research Organization (CSIRO), the genetic damage caused by deficiency of these and other nutrients (including magnesium, manganese, and vitamin E) is equivalent to or greater than the damage caused by exposure to significant doses of chemical carcinogens, ultraviolet radiation, and ionizing radiation.

In upcoming chapters, I'll detail how you can use certain foods to reduce the damage to your DNA *and* improve your DNA repair mechanisms. It's time now to take a look at our last mechanism by which eating healthier can lower your cancer risk, that of causing cancer cells to undergo a process called *differentiation.*

Diet, differentiation, and cancer risk

Differentiation is a process by which an unspecialized (stem) cell becomes a specialized cell, such as one that belongs to your heart, lung, liver, or other tissue. The process of differentiation is faulty in cancer cells, and as malignant cells rapidly grow and divide, they tend to become progressively *less* differentiated and *more* malignant. One important aim of cancer prevention and therapy involves getting these 'generic' cancer cells to differentiate into a normal cell type.

Differentiation is a worthy goal for several reasons. First, tumor cells that differentiate may reproduce more slowly. Second, they are less likely to invade other tissues. Third, the ability of these cells to undergo apoptosis may be restored. If the point of 'terminal' differentiation is reached, these cells won't multiply. "Induction of terminal differentiation means that the cancer cells are forced to behave like normal cells," explained Dr. Ivana Vucenik, an Associate Professor at the University Of Maryland School of Medicine.

The importance of differentiation in cancer treatment is taken into account by use of a grading system. In general, there are 3 grades of tumor differentiation: tumors are said to be 'well differentiated', 'moderately differentiated', or 'poorly differentiated.' Tumors classified as well differentiated contain cells that bear some degree of resemblance to the normal cells of the tissue from which they came. Clinically, the use of a grading system is important because the more differentiated a tumor is, the lesser its growth rate and the better the prognosis for a cure. Tumor differentiation also indicates response to chemotherapy. Unfortunately, what sometimes happens during chemotherapy is that the weaker, more differentiated cancer cells get weeded out. At the same time, the tougher, less differentiated ones survive, pass their hardiness on to newly created cells, and make survival more difficult for the patient. The bottom line in some cancers is that poorly differentiated tumors are associated with a decrease in survival.

A number of differentiating agents are being studied, and some of these have shown promise for achieving differentiation in ways that have low or no toxicity, unlike most forms of chemotherapy. These include inositol hexaphosphate (IP6, found in whole grains and legumes) and certain carotenoids. I'll review these in later chapters. As you read through these, you will no doubt become very impressed by the cancer-fighting power of many phytochemicals. Keep in mind however that the overriding power of an anti-cancer diet doesn't come from simply including individual foods. Your best protection is to combine a dietary pattern that provides a generous amount of all of these, while minimizing foods with pro-cancer effects, and doing both for a lifetime.

Chapter Two

Soy Foods: Your # 1 Friend in the Cancer Battle

What would you think if you found out that a certain food had a nearly miraculous ability to lower your cancer risk, but 90% of it was used to feed animals instead? Wouldn't you say that it was a poor use of our resources, especially given the incredibly high number of people affected by cancers?

The food I'm referring to is the soybean, and it's a source of phytochemicals that inhibit cancer growth in many different ways. In fact, it's hard to show that any other food has more of an anti-cancer effect. In studies with hundreds of thousands of people, eating soy foods on a regular basis has been linked with a lower risk for some of the most common cancers, including colorectal cancer, breast cancer, prostate cancer, and lung cancer. In spite of these benefits, people only consume about10% of soybeans grown in the United States. The rest is used for animal chow. This is tragic - we obviously need to eat the soybeans more than the cows do!

Thousands of studies have concluded that phytochemicals called *isoflavones* in soy foods (including soy milk, tofu, tempeh, and others) oppose cancer growth by triggering suicide (apoptosis) in cancer cells, reducing the chances a cancer will metastasize, opposing the pro-growth effect of hormones, synergistically inhibiting cancer when combined with other foods in Asian diets (for instance, certain vegetables, and green tea), and overcoming the resistance to chemotherapy drugs. These effects explain, at least to some degree, why Asian people who eat soy foods often have less cancer than Americans. Notably, the rate of these cancers increases when they move to the United states, stop consuming their traditional soy-containing diets, and start eating a Western diet.

For most of the 20th century, soybeans were not welcome on the table of the overwhelming majority of Americans. Used as animal feed for their high protein and nutrient content, they helped animals 'bulk up' faster. This allowed for a quicker entry into the slaughterhouse, and a reduction in the price of meat. As meat became cheaper, consumption increased in the U.S., followed by a number of unpleasant health consequences for the American consumer (higher blood cholesterol, weight gain, and of course, a higher cancer risk).

Although some health food stores have been carrying soy foods for many years, consumers saw the first commercially available soy food in the form of soymilk in 1996. Around the same time, patties made from soy were produced and made commercially available, intended to be a hamburger substitute for the growing number of vegetarians (and anyone else that didn't feel like eating meat every day). Since the mid-1990's, the number of soy-based meat and cheese substitutes has continued to grow, although the variety available is still far greater at specialty stores than mainstream supermarkets. This increase in the availability of soy foods seems to be gradually leading to a greater acceptance of these by the average consumer. Although it's not likely that people will give up entirely on eating meat and dairy products, a more moderate soy intake – for example, replacing cow's milk with soymilk on your breakfast cereal, and replacing meat with tofu, edamame, or tempeh a few times each week – may be enough to inhibit a key step in cancer growth. This step, which is critical for cancer cells to grow from the size of a pinhead and spread throughout your body, is called *angiogenesis*.

Soy inhibits angiogenesis

As I mentioned in Chapter 1, angiogenesis is a crucial step in cancer progression towards metastasis, which is the spread of cancer to other parts of your body, because without it, tumors would remain localized. If this were the case, surgeons could pluck them out of your body like low-hanging fruit, and you could easily survive having cancer, even repeatedly.

Let's pause for a minute and think about the implications of this. A person dies from cancer *every minute* in the United States. If you can imagine saving the majority of these people by keeping these cancers from spreading, you'll have some idea of the potential benefit anti-angiogenesis strategies have. This is unfortunately not the current state of affairs. Most cancers are found *after* they've undergone angiogenesis, which means that the treatment most people are given is palliative at best. Weapons are badly needed to prevent and obstruct angiogenesis, and this is where soy and other angiogenesis-preventing foods come in handy.

Some scientists have called soy foods "the most potent angiogenesis-inhibiting food in a plant-based diet". One of these is Dr. Fazlul Sarkar, a Professor of Pathology at Wayne State University, who has done much of the work on soy and angiogenesis. Dr. Sarkar does cancer research in conjunction with the Karmanos Cancer Institute in Detroit, and he's received grants from both the National Institutes of Health and the Department of Defense to research the effects of soy on cancer growth. His accomplishments include development of early screening tests for aggressive types of breast cancer, furthering knowledge of both cancer genes (oncogenes) and of the role of inflammation in cancer growth, adding to the knowledge of tumor suppressor genes, and the use of gene therapy for certain cancers. In spite of Dr. Sarkar's focus on basic cancer mechanisms and treatment, he stated during our interview that his interests lie mainly in cancer prevention. He and his co-workers set out to research the effect of soy on breast cancer in mid-1990. "Within two years, we showed in cell cultures that soy inhibited the growth of breast cancer cells," he began. "By 2003, we extended these findings to show that soy also inhibited breast cancer growth in animals. We also have data that shows that some of the anti-cancer phytochemicals in soy concentrate specifically in cancerous tissues," he continued. "We found that we could reduce the dose of chemotherapy in soy-fed animals by 50% and get better results on tumor killing. This is important because chemotherapy can be quite toxic."

Not surprisingly, Dr. Sarkar and his co-workers followed this by publishing research on the effect of soy in prostate cancer. One of these studies found that soy supplements reduced prostate specific antigen (PSA), an important marker of prostate cancer growth. Men with prostate cancer who received a combination of soy and lycopene (a phytochemical found in tomatoes, watermelon, and guava, discussed in Chapter Four) also experienced a reduction in PSA. They also saw and an almost 70% decrease in VEGF (vascular endothelial growth factor), a growth factor that plays a key role in angiogenesis. In another study, researchers compared giving 40 grams of either soy protein or milk protein to 58 men at high risk for developing prostate cancer.

After 6 months, significantly less men in the soy group developed prostate cancer, compared with men getting milk protein.

How does soy exert an anti-angiogenesis effect? By several mechanisms, including an influence on immune cells and the variety of chemicals they produce. "Soy inhibits inflammation," Dr. Sarkar explained. "As a result, chemicals involved in angiogenesis, like VEGF and matrix metalloproteinases, are decreased."

Stanford University researchers confirmed this effect, finding that prostate cancer-afflicted men give soy-supplemented diets experienced an effect similar to taking prescription anti-inflammatory medications. These belong to a class called NSAIDs (non-steroidal anti-inflammatory drugs). NSAIDs suppress activity of COX-2, a protein that causes inflammation, pain, and promotes cancer cell division. Interestingly, taking these drugs (aspirin is the most well known, but this group also includes ibuprofen, naprosyn, celecoxib and others) on a daily to weekly basis has been associated with a significantly lower risk of cancer deaths. They're also associated with putting a hole in your stomach lining, which could land you in the hospital with a bleeding ulcer. Half the people taking these meds regularly experience intestinal damage, and NSAID-induced GI bleeding is the 14th leading cause of death in the U.S. Put in these terms, eating more soy and other foods that suppress inflammation seems like a far more sensible anti-inflammatory strategy. Soy also inhibits growth factors that cancers need to thrive. These growth factors (EGF, FGF, IGF, VEGF and others) encourage cancers cells to divide, proliferate, and invade nearby tissues, leading to metastasis. When these growth factors can't signal a green light for cancer cell growth, they have no other choice than to go in the opposite direction, blowing themselves sky-high in a suicide-like process called apoptosis.

Soy promotes apoptosis

Apoptosis, if you remember from Chapter 1, is a process whereby cells commit hara-kiri, falling apart from within. Part of the cancer problem is that these cells lose the ability to experience apoptosis. Diet can play a cancer preventive role by restoring that ability.

In lab tests, soy phytochemicals (isoflavones) promote apoptosis by interfering with *survivin*, an anti-apoptosis protein. Survivin would normally inhibit certain proteins (enzymes called *caspases*) that are the 'wrecking ball' of apoptosis. Survivin shows up in many common cancers, and its presence is associated with a greater risk of cancer death. Isoflavones also inhibits a protein-digester called a *proteasome* that protects tumors from apoptosis, and counteracts the ability of certain growth factors to prevent apoptosis.

Similar to laboratory research, studies in isoflavone-fed animals found pro-apoptosis effects. In animals that were bred especially to serve as a model for human prostate cancer, feeding high-isoflavone soy caused a decrease in growth factors, an increase in the number of apoptotic cells, and a 40% reduction in tumor volume in just three weeks.

What about human studies? Theoretically, if an animal is bred specifically as a model for human prostate cancer, what works in animals should work in humans – i.e., apoptosis should be evident in prostate cancer-afflicted men who eat soy foods. And in one of the first studies involving men with prostate cancer, Dr. Sarkar and his colleagues at Wayne State University observed such results, obtaining clinical benefit in the form of stabilizing PSA. Other studies confirmed an increase in the 'doubling time' for PSA, an indicator of slower cancer growth.

Not all studies have revealed a cancer growth-inhibiting effect of soy alone. In fact, many of the more recently done studies have turned out to be disappointing. This shouldn't be a surprise, however. Cancers, by their very nature, are hard to beat, and if the addition of only one kind of phytochemical has a chemotherapy-like effect, it would be considered extraordinary. Studies of dietary *patterns* – usually traditional ways of eating, but also judged by how frequently people incorporate 'good-for-you foods and avoid unhealthy ones – have revealed more of an effect on markers of prostate cancer growth. For instance, the superior cancer-fighting ability of a traditional Japanese diet was obvious when comparing two groups of Japanese men (one native, the other 'Americanized') being treated for prostate cancer. As expected with a traditional Japanese diet, the amount of soy breakdown products in the urine of the native men was also much higher than in the Americanized Japanese. The Westernized group had (not surprisingly) significantly higher levels of body fat and blood fats. More importantly, an apoptosis-inducing caspase was expressed more in the native Japanese than in their Western counterparts.

Soy foods also have more of a dynamic anti-cancer effect when combined with other foods high in anti-cancer phytochemicals. So far, researchers have documented growth-inhibiting effects on prostate cancers when soy was combined with tomato products and with curcumin, an anti-inflammatory phytochemical found in turmeric spice. Only one clinical trial utilized a combination approach, combining soy with a low-fat diet, vitamin E, selenium and multivitamins, but the effects were more dynamic. These included reductions in growth factors and PSA, along with lowering the amount of available testosterone. The importance of reducing the presence of testosterone can't be understated, for a number of reasons. First, because removing the growth-promoting impact of hormones (testosterone and estrogen) is known to promote apoptosis. Second, anti-estrogen and anti-testosterone treatments are a standard part of therapy for both breast and prostate cancers. It is to the impact of soy on hormones then that we should now turn.

Soy opposes cancer-promoting hormones

Hormone-related cancers are some of the most common types of malignancy. In fact, if breast and prostate cancers alone were taken out of the picture, up to 45% of the total cancer burden would be eliminated. This would undoubtedly save of millions of lives, in addition to *billions* in health care dollars. What seems very curious (and what should greatly trouble the mind of both laypersons and researchers, but seems not to) is the fact that these two cancers were relatively uncommon just a few decades ago. The steep rise in both these cancers has to a great extent paralleled the obesity epidemic, abandoning of traditional diets, and the exposure of an entire nation to a diet high in animal products and refined carbohydrates.

One of many scientists working on connections between soy intake, hormones, and cancer risk is Dr. Joseph Zhou, an Assistant Professor of Surgery at Harvard's Beth Israel Deaconess

Medical Center. Although his title might lead you to think he spends most of his time slicing and dicing, he actually takes a large chunk of it to do research on cancer prevention. "In general, my research focuses on the role of dietary components in the prevention of cancers, including breast cancer, prostate cancer, and bladder cancer," Dr. Zhou began. "My work has focused on the anti-cancer activities of soy and green tea. We use a variety of approaches - basic lab techniques, cell cultures, and animal models - to figure out the possible mechanisms," he continued.

Dr. Zhou's research is based on an ever-increasing number of population studies that have shown a high intake of soy foods is associated with a lower risk for two major types of hormone-related cancers (breast and prostate cancers). Breast cancer risk appears to be reduced when women regularly eat soy foods, although there is some disagreement among scientists about whether this is an effect of soy itself or soy foods within the context of an Asian-style diet. For example, studies have shown that other foods in the Japanese diet (edible seaweed, for example) can reduce the amount of available estrogen, which could help lower breast cancer risk. "Some studies show that certain phytochemicals inhibit estrogen-dependent breast cancer by affecting estrogen receptor-related signaling pathways," commented Dr. Zhou. "The main mechanism is probably the phytoestrogens competing with estrogen for binding to estrogen receptors, the same as the drug Tamoxifen® - but this again is just one part of the possible mechanisms."

Eating soy foods regularly is also thought to lower the risk for prostate cancer. Importantly, soy is associated with a lower risk for developing 'aggressive' prostate cancer, the more life-threatening kind than the slow-growing type many men have. The distinction between having *any* kind of cancer and an *aggressively-growing* type is an important one: having prostate cancer is not the same thing as dying from it, and mortality from this cancer is ten times lower in Asian countries than in the West.

Isoflavones also reduce prostate cancer risk by increasing the liver's production of sex hormone-binding globulin (SHBG), which ties up some of the free testosterone floating around in the blood and getting into the prostate. "Isoflavones in soy, and certain phytochemicals in green tea, can also inhibit the [5-AR] enzyme that converts testosterone to dihydrotestosterone (DHT)," Dr. Zhou added. 5-AR produces a form of testosterone (DHT) that appears to increase prostate cancer growth by sticking to the hormone receptor more than testosterone itself does, an effect which magnifies the hormone-triggering effect on cancer growth. Asian men who have lower prostate cancer risk than their Western counterparts make less DHT, so this effect may be one of the most important ones in prostate cancer prevention.

Soy prevents cancer cell proliferation

Stopping the process of cancer cell proliferation is a goal of cancer treatment, one so important that many scientists have dedicated their careers to it. Given its importance and the fact that diet has turned out to be an important influence on proliferation, it makes sense that we should take some time to know more about it.

But what *is* 'cell proliferation'? Taking the root of the word *proliferate* as a partial explanation, we see that it contains the words *pro* and *life* – literally, more life, the creation of more cells.

Most cells in the body proliferate, or reproduce, at various rates (think of skin cells, which do so constantly, and immune cells, which proliferate at faster rates during an infection). With cancer cells, proliferation is deregulated, often occurring at faster rates than in most normal cells. Proliferation occurs through a process called mitosis. Like a bicycle wheel that needs energy to turn and a rider to provide the energy, the cell cycle needs certain proteins to work in order to accomplish mitosis and make more cancer cells. These proteins include *tyrosine kinases* (TKs), *cyclins*, and *cyclin-dependent kinases* (CDKs).

Cancer cells, like other types of cells, also need a sort of molecular 'stamp of approval' that conditions are right for mitosis to occur. Malignant cells get the go-ahead to divide when a message is passed down from the outside of the cells to the cell's interior, in a series of steps called *signal transduction*. You might think of it as a process similar to the chain of command needed for dropping a bomb, involving a commanding officer that gives the order to a lower-ranking officer, who radios the airman that delivers it on a target. In the case of dividing cancer cells, the commanding officer comes in the form of growth factors and certain chemicals (cytokines) the immune system creates. Diet influences the creation of these mitosis-encouraging proteins, allowing for cancer growth or prevention. Importantly, soy foods and other dietary compounds have the ability to inhibit both these proteins and the actual phases of mitosis.

One of the earliest-discovered anti-cancer effects of soy was genistein's ability to inhibit TKs. During a telephone conversation I had with Dr. Sarkar, he pointed out some additional ways in which soy phytochemicals work against cancer cell proliferation. One of these results in inhibiting a cyclin-CDK partnership that would normally help cancer cells to proliferate. "Genistein significantly increases a CDK inhibitor called p21/WAF1," Dr. Sarkar began." That is the most consistent data so far. However, we also found that genistein causes the cell cycle to stop at the G2/M phase by down-regulating cyclin B1. If you don't have cyclin B1, it means the cell cycle isn't going to progress."

A good look at the laboratory studies that detail soy's specific anti-cell cycle effects help to explain why it is associated with lowering the risk for many cancers. One of these effects is inhibition of *epidermal growth factor* (EGF), a TK that drives cell proliferation "Genistein decreases activity of the EGF receptor and several kinase enzymes, and decreases signal transduction," Dr. Sarkar explained. "In fact, it down-regulates the whole pathway from the cell surface receptor to the nucleus."

Soy and differentiation

Differentiation is a process by which an unspecialized (stem) cell becomes a specialized cell: one that belongs to your heart, lung, liver, muscle, or other tissue. As I discussed in chapter One, the process of differentiation is faulty in cancer cells, and as malignant cells rapidly grow and divide, they tend to become progressively less differentiated and more malignant. An important goal of cancer prevention and therapy involves getting these 'generic' cancer cells to differentiate to a normal type. If differentiation is achieved, tumor cells may reproduce more slowly, become less likely to invade other tissues, and regain the ability for apoptosis. If the point of 'terminal' differentiation is reached, these cells won't multiply at all. "Induction of terminal differentiation means that the cancer cells are forced to behave like normal cells," explained Dr. Ivana Vucenik, an Associate Professor at the University Of Maryland School of Medicine. A number of differentiating agents are being studied, and some of these have shown promise for achieving differentiation in ways that have low or no toxicity, unlike most forms of chemotherapy.

The importance of differentiation in cancer treatment is taken into account by use of a grading system. In general, there are 3 grades of tumor differentiation: tumors are said to be 'well differentiated', 'moderately differentiated', or 'poorly differentiated'. Tumors classified as well differentiated contain cells that bear some degree of resemblance to the normal cells of the tissue from which they came. Clinically, the use of a grading system is important because the more differentiated a tumor is, the less is its growth rate and the better the prognosis for a cure. Tumor differentiation also indicates response to chemotherapy. Unfortunately, what sometimes happens during chemotherapy is that the weaker, more differentiated cancer cells get weeded out. At the same time, tougher, less differentiated ones survive, pass their hardiness on to newly created cells, and make survival more difficult for the patient. The bottom line in some cancers is that poorly differentiated tumors are associated with a decrease in survival.

Evidence of an effect of soy foods on differentiation began in 1990 with the efforts of Dr. Andreas Constantinou, a University of Cyprus biochemist. Dr. Constantinou and his co-workers discovered that genistein causes differentiation, and proceeded to work out the pathways by which it does so in human breast cancer cells. Dr. Coral Lamartiniere, a Cancer Center Senior Scientist currently with the University of Alabama's Department of Pharmacology and Toxicology, further built upon Dr. Constantinou's work. He and his co-workers have been studying the role of environmental chemicals that girls and young women are exposed to, and how these chemicals and genistein may impact the risk for breast cancer. Dr. Lamartiniere explained the relationships between phytochemicals in soy and differentiation during a phone conversation, shortly after the publication of studies he and his colleagues had performed.

"The mechanism of genistein's protection against breast cancer is related to differentiation of the mammary gland," he began. "There's a comparison to be made with what happens in humans during puberty and pregnancy, when differentiation of the mammary gland occurs due to an increase in hormones. Genistein reduces the number of what are called 'terminal end buds -' a part of the mammary gland that are less differentiated and more susceptible to chemical carcinogens," he continued. "Genistein also increased the number of lobules, a part of the gland that is most differentiated and *least* susceptible to cancer-causing chemicals."

Dr. Lamartiniere cautioned that the timing of exposure to genistein is a deciding factor in whether soy foods induce differentiation. "The critical period for genistein exposure is the early post-natal period for rats, which is equivalent to adolescence in human beings," he detailed. "In fact, there's evidence from two population studies that show soy foods protect against breast cancer most when girls are exposed to these near puberty, at roughly ages 10 to 12."

Although many growth factors are linked to cancer risk, Dr. Lamartiniere found in his genistein-treated animals that the timing at which these peak in the blood were a more important factor than their presence alone. If animals were given genistein *early* in life, it *increased* certain growth factors, stimulated differentiation, and reduced the number of cells in the mammary gland. As a result, these animals experienced a *decrease* in these growth factors and a lower risk for breast cancer later in life. "In these animals, the mammary gland produced more casein, a protein indicating milk production," Dr. Lamartiniere elaborated. "This is another bit of evidence that differentiation had occurred."

In male animals fed genistein-fortified chow, Dr. Lamartiniere and his co-workers found that a significantly lower number had poorly differentiated prostate cancer than those given normal food. More importantly, these effects occurred in animals *at blood levels comparable to those found in humans who habitually eat soy foods.* This kind of effect isn't often shown for phytochemicals, and is a critical step in documenting the possibility that a certain food will have meaningful, anti-cancer effects if people make a habit of eating it.

Soy foods also affect differentiation by activating certain receptors ('peroxisome proliferator activated receptors', or PPARs) that are the target of certain drugs for diabetes. Soybeans are also a great dietary source of *sphingolipids*, which are fats found in the membranes of all our body cells, especially brain and nerve tissues. Breakdown products of sphingolipids called *ceramides* play roles in tumor differentiation, as well as other aspects of cancer prevention (for example, growth inhibition and induction of apoptosis).

Soy and detoxification

Soy foods can lower your cancer risk by affecting the body's detoxification system in two different ways. First, using soy as a protein source doesn't carry the same toxic burden that meats do. Second, soy phytochemicals may influence Phase I detoxification enzymes, the kind that affect both activation of carcinogens and hormones involved in cancer risk.

Remembering back to the earlier explanation of detoxification, you may recall that *lowering* the activity of certain detox pathways are an important way the body prevents activation of pro-carcinogens. Researchers were able to show that soy could affect this pathway, by experimenting with a potential carcinogen (DMBA, which depends on Phase I activation to do its dirty work) in two groups of cancer cells. To one group, soy isoflavones were added, and both sets were looked at to see to what degree DMBA-DNA adducts (a cancer marker) were formed. A high amount of DMBA-DNA adducts would be expected, and a lower amount would be a key indicator that soy was having a protective effect. As expected, Phase I enzymes activated DMBA and caused formation of DMBA-DNA adducts. However, results clearly showed that the soy isoflavones inhibited the Phase I enzymes, prevented a change in DMBA from a potential to a full-blown carcinogen, and protected against DNA damage.

The ability of soy to inhibit Phase I enzymes that impact hormones is another example of how isoflavones affect cancer risk. I spoke with Dr. Heidi Cross, an investigator from the University of Vienna's Medical School, where she was doing research in this area. Dr. Cross's research focused on interactions between soy and vitamin D. At the time we spoke, Dr. Cross and her colleagues had published evidence that soy phytochemicals could prevent Phase I enzymes from breaking down the active form of vitamin D. This nutrient, which is also known as a hormone, is known to have important anti-cancer effects, particularly with regard to colon, rectum, and breast cancers. The Phase I enzyme that breaks down the active, anti-cancer form of vitamin D is increasingly active in the colon as cancer progresses, and its inhibition by soy may represent yet another important means by which soy renders an anti-cancer effect.

In spite of all these efforts to reveal soy's anti-cancer mechanisms and the numerous studies revealing a benefit to the prevention of cancer, a great deal of opposition remains to eating soy foods. I'll reveal both sides of the argument below, and you can decide for yourself whether eating or avoiding soy is a wiser anti-cancer strategy.

The soy-estrogen-breast cancer controversy: the anti-soy argument

After having spoken to individuals and groups regarding soy foods and breast cancer risk over the past few years, it's become obvious that a significant number of women are reticent ('frightened' would be a better word) about eating soy foods. And a portion of the scientific and clinical community is to blame for what could be properly called 'soy paranoia'. The controversy stems from the fact that a significant percentage of breast cancers are estrogen-related, and some phytochemicals in soy are also estrogens, albeit *plant* estrogens ('phytoestrogens', not the same as human estrogen). With respect to soy foods, 'guilt by association' appears to have occurred, and by golly, if a food has estrogen in it, and estrogen causes breast cancer, then that food should be avoided. Right?

Not exactly.

There is no straightforward relationship between any and all types of estrogen and breast cancer risk. The links between *plant* sources of estrogen and risk for breast cancer turn out to be even less clear that these are harmful. In fact, soy phytoestrogens actually compete with the body's own estrogen, resulting in antagonism of the growth-promoting effects of this hormone on cancer cells.

The small body of evidence indicating that eating soy foods have estrogenic effects come from laboratory studies of estrogen receptor positive breast cancer cells isolated in a soupy growth medium, and from a limited number of studies in humans. In the former, phytoestrogens increased the number of breast cancer cells and reversed the anti-cancer effect of tamoxifen, an estrogen antagonist.

Unfortunately, many physicians, oncologists included, jumped on the anti-soy bandwagon, ignoring the larger body of data on the safety of soy foods. Many is the time I've heard a woman say, "My Doctor told me not to eat soy" if she was at risk for, or had been in remission from, breast cancer.

There are several problems with this advice, beginning with the fact that physicians aren't nutritionists. As an Internist friend of mine often points out, our Docs get just *one* class on nutrition during their entire medical school education. This borders on the insane, given that poor diet is the basis for the overwhelming majority of diseases patients see physicians for. As to why people believe this advice, I can only speculate that we as a society have the misguided notion that physicians know everything. As any physician herself will tell you, they don't, which is why they frequently refer patients to other practitioners, whether they be other physicians, physical therapists, mental health professionals, or nutritionists. However, if your Doc gives you nutrition advice without taking the time to read the body of literature on a topic (something very few take the time to do), the results may be the opposite of what either of you wants.

A main reason for ignoring advice to avoid soy has to do with the alternatives. If not soy protein, what other protein choices are left that are compatible with lower cancer risk? Anyone who advises women to avoid soy will by default be suggesting that they continue to eat animal foods for protein, because few will confine their protein intake to plant sources. Yet animal proteins are the very same foods that can increase cancer growth. Even including *some* soy protein in our diets leaves space for other protein sources; however, these should come from foods that lower, rather than raise cancer risk (for instance, other legumes, nuts/seeds, and fish). Protein *choices* aside, a basic problem with protein still exists, which is that Americans are overly focused on the intake of this nutrient, building meals around it in spite of the fact that it represents the lowest amount of calories (15% or less) that we need.

Why the anti-soy argument doesn't hold up

Arguments against eating soy fall into several categories. The first concerns the potentially estrogenic effect of soy. This point may be written off as a non-issue if we consider that pharmacologic doses of estrogen used for hormone replacement therapy have not been clearly demonstrated to increase breast cancer risk (although combining estrogen with progesterone does). In other words, how can the estrogenic effect of soy represent a cancer risk when high doses of estrogen itself don't?

One of the most outspoken proponents of soy foods is Dr. Mark Messina, an Associate Professor of Nutrition at Loma Linda University. In a summary article co-authored with Dr. Charles Wood of Wake Forest University's Dept. of Pathology, Drs. Messina and Wood took a critical look at the studies that seemed to indicate undesirable effects of eating soy foods. According to their analysis, many of these studies had design flaws that make it unreasonable to base recommendations for humans on. In two of these in which an estrogenic effect was suspected, both lacked a control group, and found that the undesired (i.e., estrogenic) effect existed both at baseline and far beyond the point when these women stopped eating soy foods.

A second flaw concerns what could be called the 'saccharin argument.' Studies of rodents who developed mammary cancers were fed 5 times the amount of phytoestrogens found in traditional soy foods, much the same as when rodents who developed bladder cancer were fed doses of saccharin and cyclamates much greater than humans would be exposed to. No one takes this kind of evidence seriously anymore (or at least, they shouldn't).

There are still other arguments in favor of not being afraid of soy. Two studies in women given isolated soy protein or textured vegetable protein (not soy foods like tofu, soy milk, or tempeh) found an increase in nipple fluid aspirate, indicating an estrogen-like response to the soy feeding. While these results were reported as evidence of an estrogenic effect, the media failed to report that more recent studies revealed no increase in nipple fluid aspirate in women fed two servings per day of soy foods for six months. Another marker of estrogen exposure and breast cancer risk, that of breast density, was found not affected by soy intake, according to UK researchers who reviewed eight studies involving nearly 1,300 women.

The pro-soy argument

Nearly all published scientific evidence of soy foods on breast cancer show that women eating the most isoflavones have a 5% to 20% lower risk, compared to women eating the least amount. Perhaps the most convincing evidence of the benefits of soy on breast cancer risk comes from studies of women who have already had breast cancer and are fighting to survive. One of these is the Shanghai Breast Cancer Survival Study, in which more than 5,000 female breast cancer survivors were examined to determine the impact of soy foods on breast cancer outcome. The researchers concluded that the women who ate the most soy had a roughly 30% lower risk for dying from breast cancer, compared to women eating the least amount. In Shanghai, intake of soy is much greater than the U.S.; nevertheless, another study of 1,954 breast cancer survivors in the U.S. also was suggestive of a protective association between soy and breast cancer, even with much lower average intake. In this study, intake of soy phytochemicals appeared to reduce the risk for breast cancer recurrence. Interestingly, both these studies found that soy had a complimentary anti-cancer effect with tamoxifen, an anti-estrogen drug. Laboratory studies explain why this is so. While estrogen causes cancer growth by stimulating estrogen receptor alpha (ERα), phytoestrogens stimulate a different type of estrogen receptor (ERβ). This receptor actually binds with phytoestrogens to a much greater degree (up to 5 times higher) than estrogen does, inhibits cell proliferation, and triggers apoptosis.

A less scientific (but far more practical) argument for eating more soy has to do with where our protein intake should come from. High fat meats, eggs, and whole milk dairy products (e.g., cheese) have too much saturated fat and cholesterol to be considered safe. Lower fat versions of these foods (egg whites, nonfat dairy products, low fat meats) are one alternative, but none of these foods has the antioxidant phytochemicals or fiber Americans badly need to lower cancer risk. At best, they should be used sparingly. This leaves other legumes and nuts as protein sources. These are both very nutritious, but have certain problems in everyday use. Legumes have very limited acceptance among most Americans; we can be honest here and say without a doubt that the 'flatulence factor' is a major reason. Nuts have the advantage of greater consumer acceptance, but Americans also eat them more rarely, perhaps because of concern over allergy or their high calorie density. Fish consumption has experienced a resurgence due to an increased awareness of the benefits of omega-3 fats, but the number of times each week that a person can eat fish is usually limited by the expense or the lack of time needed to prepare it. Variety is good, but moderation requires that we get less protein from animal sources and more from plants. When Americans learn how to do this, it will represent a giant leap forward in our ability to lower cancer risk and create better health in general.

Chapter Three

Green tea: The All-Hulk, No-Bulk Cancer Fighter

In nearly every place I've lived, a Starbucks has been built, or was already there by the time I moved in. Certain cities had not just one, but also two, three, or even *four* coffee shops, all within a five-mile drive. To be sure, coffee is incredibly popular; maybe this has to do with the ever-increasing number of things one can do to and with coffee: iced coffee, cappuccino, latte, espresso, and coffee drinks flavored with syrups, just to name a few. Coffee is actually good for you, in moderate amounts, with the exception of people who are sensitive to its' stimulant effects (and people like me, who get raging heartburn from it – unfortunately). There's even some data indicating it may help lower the risk for cancers of the liver, endometrium, colon and rectum. Even so, if you want to lower your cancer risk, the evidence says that green tea is a far stronger, bigger, and better weapon against cancer.

Tea, it has been said, is the most popular beverage in the world, next to water. During the time I spent reviewing research and interviewing scientists regarding their work on green tea, it became apparent to me that the potential for this beverage to inhibit cancer growth is truly amazing. Importantly, the phytochemicals in green tea - each with a name harder to pronounce than the last (*epicatechin* (EC), *epicatechin gallate* (ECG), *epigallocatechin* (EGC), and *epigallocatechin gallate* (EGCG) - do so in ways that are similar to drugs, but without the toxicity. And once the word gets out about how powerful an anti-cancer effect it has, it wouldn't be surprising if 'tea houses' became as common on our landscape as coffee shops currently are. In fact, it's already starting to happen.

I began by interviewing Dr. Mohsen Meydani, a Senior Scientist at the USDA's Human Nutrition Research Center on Aging. Dr. Meydani is actually more known for having done landmark work on the importance of vitamin E on immune function. In late 1997 however, he and his lab partners turned their attention to green tea. "One of my graduate students and I were working on a green tea phytochemical called EGCG and how it affected atherosclerosis in animals," he began. Dr. Meydani and his student noticed that old-fashioned hydrogen peroxide could stimulate angiogenesis, and found that EGCG could prevent this process. "The effect was quite dramatic, actually," he continued. "We reduced the dose of EGCG considerably and still saw these effects. "EGCG doesn't just prevent angiogenesis by its antioxidant effect. It prevents a whole series of steps that lead to angiogenesis," he concluded.

Soon after Dr. Meydani's lab began work on green tea, Dr. Spiridione Garbisa, a Professor of Histology at Italy's University of Padova Medical School, began his own investigation. Dr. Garbisa is a prolific researcher, and a co-discoverer of the protein enzymes called *matrix metalloproteinases* (MMP) that are key to the ability of cancer cells to invade nearby tissues and create metastasis.

I asked Dr. Garbisa how he got interested in green tea and angiogenesis. "I read a one-page communication in [the scientific journal] *Nature* from a former collaborator of Dr. Folkman's lab," he began. "This scientist reported that angiogenesis was inhibited by drinking tea, and that the active compound was a molecule called EGCG, very abundant in green tea. I was already aware that certain protein enzymes were involved in angiogenesis, tumor invasion, and metastasis," he continued. "The idea came to me that the prevention of what these enzymes do might be the result of inhibition by EGCG."

Finding inhibitors of angiogenesis has obvious significance for cancer treatment. However, such research is expensive, generally coming from the deep pockets of drug companies who expect the strong possibility of a huge payoff. Still, there's also no guarantee that *if* angiogenesis inhibitors were found, they would be effective for interfering with cancer growth without being toxic to the host. The finding that green tea phytochemicals throw a monkey wrench into angiogenesis was therefore a big deal to the cancer research community. You might imagine the surprised look on the faces of many scientists, as their colleagues came to them with such news after they'd spent months screening hundreds of chemicals for angiogenesis inhibition: (*"TEA? You've got to be kidding. This is a joke, right?"*)

Green tea has turned out to be only one of many food-based angiogenesis inhibitors. Even so, preventing angiogenesis in lab tests or in animals doesn't necessarily translate to therapeutic effects in humans. An additional hurdle must be overcome: the active phytochemicals must be available in human blood or tissue at levels high enough to affect cancer growth, which can be hard to prove. So it was all the more exciting when Dr. Garbisa's research found that these levels might be attainable in humans. "The results we got confirmed that the enzymes involved in angiogenesis and metastasis are very effectively blunted by EGCG, at concentrations not much higher than those measured in the serum of moderate green-tea drinkers," Dr. Garbisa emphasized. "It's already been reported that EGCG also boosts the beneficial effects of tamoxifen, an anti-cancer drug for breast cancer. EGCG could become an anti-cancer drug in itself," he added. "Some synthetic inhibitors are more powerful than EGCG in laboratory experiments, but in animals and humans they present heavy side effects, for which reason most of them have been abandoned. Green tea and EGCG are safe and very well tolerated, even at high doses." Dr. Vaqar Adhami, an Associate Scientist from the University of Wisconsin Medical School's Department of Dermatology, came to similar conclusions. "Although EGCG is weaker than drugs that inhibit angiogenesis, it's safer, and can be used in larger doses without worrying about side-effects," he opined.

I spoke with Dr. Adhami about research he and his colleagues had published on the impact of green tea on prostate and skin cancers. "We discovered around year 2000 that EGCG reduces levels of IGF-1, which has been linked to many cancers," Dr. Adhami noted. Dr. Hasan Mukhtar, a Professor of Dermatology and colleague of Dr. Adhami, elaborated further. "IGF levels return to normal when animals are given green tea to drink," he began. "We don't know for sure that this occurs in tumors in humans; we need to do more research," he cautioned.

Dr. Adhami and his colleagues also published evidence that green tea phytochemicals inhibit metalloproteinases. "It was around October of November of 2002 that we discovered EGCG could inhibit these enzymes," Dr. Adhami recalled. "We also showed that in a mouse model, the human equivalent of four cups a day of green tea was almost completely effective in blocking the progress of prostate cancer."

In addition to restraining angiogenesis, phytochemicals in green tea also help trigger the event known as apoptosis, which is known to be an important goal of cancer treatment.

Green tea promotes suicide in cancerous cells

Apoptosis is, as I described in Chapter I, is a form of 'programmed' cell death. While reading studies on the links between diet and cancer through apoptosis, I ran across publications by a Rutgers University scientist named Chung Yang. As a Professor and Chairperson in the Department of Chemical Biology, Dr. Yang and his colleagues performed several studies that helped to explain how green tea promotes apoptosis. When I spoke with Dr. Yang, he introduced a discussion of his work by referring to the role of growth factors in cancer. Where green tea really shines, according to Dr. Yang, is in its ability to block not just one, but also *several* of these growth factors. Dr. Yang described the effect of green tea on a growth factor that is especially important due to its ability to inhibit apoptosis. He and his colleagues found that the phytochemical EGCG in green tea inactivates the receptor for EGF in cell cultures, and that apoptosis was enhanced in lung tumors of experimental animals given green tea in their drinking water. The question that followed was obvious: does green tea reduce these anti-apoptosis growth factors and lower cancer risk in humans? Both population studies and clinical research seem to give it the thumbs up here. A study of more than 42,000 Japanese men found that those who drank green tea throughout the day (5 cups' worth) had half the risk for developing advanced prostate cancer, compared with men who didn't drink the stuff. Two clinical trials appear to bear out the benefits seen in epidemiological studies. In the first of these, men with a pre-cancerous prostate condition who took a green tea extract were significantly protected against developing prostate cancer, compared to men not taking the supplement. The second, a study conducted by researchers at the Louisiana State University Health Sciences Center with men suffering from prostate cancer, revealed that a green tea concentrate does in fact significantly decrease not only IGF-1, but other growth factors (HGF, VEGF) involved in cancer growth, along with prostate-specific antigen (PSA, a well-know marker of cancer growth). And studies at the prestigious Mayo Clinic's Division of Hematology found that green tea also appears to inhibit the growth of leukemia cells. These results were found in a very small number of patients; however, they give further weight to the finding in Asian populations of an inverse risk for leukemia in persons who drink more green tea, compared with non-tea drinkers.

Another way green tea helps trigger apoptosis is by blocking an enzyme (fatty acid synthase, FAS) that cancer cells use for their growth and survival. FAS is associated with a poor prognosis in many cancers, and scientists have found that blocking FAS is an effective way to kill cancer cells. This is good news for individuals with higher FAS levels, which show up particularly in hormone-related malignancies (breast and prostate cancers). A woman's chances of dying from breast cancer are four times greater if she's found to have high FAS levels; in men with prostate cancer, the chances are four times greater that disease recurrence will result if FAS levels are high. In patients with colon cancer, FAS levels are associated with the severity of the cancer stage, and patients with the more life-threatening Stage III and IV cancers have much more FAS in their blood than do patients with Stage I and II cancers.

Other than green tea, several other phytochemicals commonly found in many fruits and vegetables (quercetin, luteolin, apigenin, kaempferol) and olive oil also inhibit FAS in certain types of cancer cells, as do omega-3 fatty acids and a kind of fat found in evening primrose oil. However, these effects have only been shown in the lab, not in humans, so we don't yet know if eating these would result in an anti-cancer effect.

Green tea: stops the cycle, kills the cyclist, and dismantles the wheels

Phytochemicals in green tea interfere with cancer cell proliferation by down-regulating cyclins, suppressing CDKs, and up-regulating CDK inhibitors, the net result of which is apoptosis. Dr. Vaqar Adhami and his colleagues also found that EGCG arrests cells in the G0/G1 phase. Importantly, EGCG up-regulates a critical CDK inhibitor ('WAF/p21') in both testosterone-sensitive and the tougher-to-kill testosterone-*insensitive* types of prostate cancer cells that are more likely to result in death from this cancer. EGCG, they suggested, might actually be imposing an 'artificial cell cycle checkpoint,' the kind that is usually missing in cancer cells and would, in a healthy organism, order the cell to stop mitosis or commit apoptosis.

Dr. I. Bernard Weinstein, a scientist with Columbia University's Institute of Human Nutrition, spoke with me before his death regarding his work on green tea, summarizing evidence that green tea stops the cell cycle at just about every step. Green tea first reduces IGF-1 availability to cancer cells, and then inhibits the tyrosine kinase enzymes that get kick-started by growth factors like IGF and EGF. Green tea phytochemicals also increases the levels of the tumor suppressor p53.

Enthusiasm for using green tea for cancer prevention, as any scientists worthy of his diploma will tell you, has to come from evidence other than studies performed in the laboratory and in small animals, neither of which are guaranteed to apply to humans with cancer. However, with green tea, the evidence is fairly strong that what Drs. Adhami, Weinstein, and others have found in the lab does apply to humans. Studies in men at risk for prostate cancer due to having a pre-cancerous condition (high grade prostatic intraepithelial neoplasia, HGPIN) found that green tea extract reduced the incidence of prostate cancer development from 9 men (30% of the placebo group) to 1 person (3%) in the group taking the tea extract. Another study on the effects of green tea in prostate cancer compared Japanese men who drank 5 cups of green tea per day with men drinking less than 1 cup per day. Although the diagnosis of *localized* prostate cancer wasn't altered by tea drinking in these men, the higher tea consumers had roughly half the risk for developing *advanced* prostate cancer. This evidence was made stronger by a UCLA study in which pathologists asked men who were scheduled for prostate removal to drink a large amount (about 48 ounces) of either green or black tea or soda each day for five days. Researchers performed a prostate biopsy, measured the amounts of tea phytochemicals (EGC, EC, EGCG, and ECG) in the prostate post-surgery, and incubated prostate cancer cells with blood serum from the tea and cola drinkers. The UCLA pathologists were able to show, for the first time, that green tea phytochemicals actually were present in the prostate. More importantly, they were able to show that the blood of tea drinkers significantly reduced proliferation in prostate cancer cells, while the blood of cola drinkers did not.

Practically speaking, drinking green tea is a cheap and enjoyable way to lower your cancer risk. There are many flavors to choose from, and decaffeinated versions are available for those who want to avoid a stimulant effect. It makes fairly good iced tea, although I prefer to brew mine with black tea blended in, for a stronger tea flavor. It's also a simpler form of cancer risk reduction, because all you need is hot water – no lengthy food preparation is involved. The only caveat is that you need to drink four to five cups per day. However, that sort of diligence can pay off in a major way over the long haul, so it's worth the effort.

Chapter Four

Attack of the Killer Tomatoes – and Beyond

The word 'carotenoids' should make you think of carrots, which is a clue to how these phyto-chemicals are identified. Carotenoids are pigments that make sweet potatoes orange, mangos yellow, tomatoes red, pink grapefruits pink, and vegetables like broccoli and spinach green. Although a few can be converted in the body to vitamin A, their importance goes far beyond this role; their main health benefits seem to be with regard to cancer prevention.

Carotenoids are the pop music stars of nutrients, reinventing their own importance every several years as data emerge on their importance. Most baby-boomers remember hearing as children "carrots are good for your eyes," and some can still recite numerous quotes from Bugs Bunny, the carrot-chewing cartoon icon who served as a reminder of this age-old wisdom. The importance of the (alpha- and beta-) carotenes to eye health eventually faded in the minds of consumers. However, after a number of studies revealed a possible cancer-preventive effect of this nutrient (circa 1980), it was replaced by a new trend: taking beta-carotene supplements. After it became apparent roughly 14 years later that taking a pill every day couldn't achieve the same cancer-preventing benefit as a lifetime of healthy eating (surprise, surprise), carotenoids again disappeared from the public view... but not for long.

Just one year later, Harvard researchers published a study revealing that foods containing the carotenoid *lycopene* might reduce cancer risk (specifically, prostate cancer). This was followed by a slew of other studies on lycopene and cancer risk, many of which confirmed the Harvard team's findings. In spite of hopeful data from studies in cell cultures, animals, and human populations, the Food and Drug Administration (FDA) concluded in 2007 there was "no credible evidence" tying either lycopene or tomatoes (the chief source of lycopene in most American's diets) to the risk for cancers of the prostate, lung, colon and rectum, GI tract, breast, ovaries, endometrium, cervix or pancreas. Reviews by other scientists were in disagreement with FDA's conclusions, particularly concerning prostate cancer. Since the FDA review was published, many additional studies have been published linking higher lycopene intakes to lower cancer risk. And many studies have, not unexpectedly, come to the opposite conclusion.

Carotenoids are, as a group, undoubtedly involved in cancer prevention, although whether or not they do so *when separated from the foods they are in* is still being investigated. These controversies drive certain scientists bonkers, as I found out when talking with Dr. T. Colin Campbell, a Professor Emeritus of Nutritional Biochemistry at Cornell University. Dr. Campbell is author of *The China Study*, the conclusions of which can be summed up in a short sentence: plant-based diets lower cancer risk, and animal foods increase cancer rates. When hearing the topic of my book, Dr. Campbell expressed great concern that I might be writing about the virtues of phytochemicals alone. Although I could not tape the interview in this case (we met at a cancer conference by accident) Dr. Campbell's message was clear: the ability of a plant-based to lower cancer risk is an intrinsic combination of fiber, vitamins, minerals, phytochemicals, plant protein, and a lack of saturated fat and cholesterol found in animal foods. It's extremely unlikely, say he and other supporters of this position, that a single vitamin, mineral, phytochemical, or any other component of a plant-based diet will be revealed as a 'magic bullet' for cancer, when separated from the foods they're contained in. It's the interaction between these - 'synergy', as some call it - that accounts for the total protective effect. We Nutritionists are nearly completely (if not entirely) in agreement here. And many scientists are gradually realizing that a single ingredient, 'reductionist' approach to investigating phytochemicals doesn't do justice to the subtle, overlapping ways that foods help prevent cancer. Yet the overwhelming number of researchers continues to try and isolate single ingredients and use these in a 'magic bullet'-like fashion.

How carotenoids work to lower cancer risk

Reductionist approaches aside, when scientists do what they do – which is, rendering down the active components of a substance to find out what makes it tick – we get valuable clues to how foods protect us, which can be used to make recommendations as to what we should eat. So far, the evidence obtained from lab studies shows that carotenoid-containing foods help lower cancer risk by activating detoxification pathways, interfering with growth factors, triggering apoptosis, opposing proliferation, stimulating immunity, helping to repair DNA, and triggering differentiation. I'll discuss these mechanisms below, with commentary from a number of scientists I spoke with who have done groundbreaking work in this area.

Carotenoids activate detoxification enzymes

Phase II detoxification enzymes work to reduce cancer risk in part by making foreign chemicals water-soluble. However, they first need to be switched on, and this occurs through what's called an *Antioxidant Response Element* (ARE). The ARE also turns on other protective antioxidant enzymes, ones that combat the free radicals that contribute to cancer and most other diseases.

I spoke with Dr. Joseph Levy of Israel's Ben-Gurion University about work he and his colleagues performed on the ARE. "Put simply, when you have toxins or carcinogens attacking our cells, our bodies turn on this [ARE] system," Dr. Levy began. "It produces a lot of enzymes which convert toxins and carcinogens that can cause potentially cancer-causing DNA mutations to less toxic forms."

Dr. Levy and others in his lab were aware of data showing that one of the anti-cancer benefits of eating carotenoid-containing fruits and vegetables was an increase in Phase II enzymes. Very close to the time we spoke on the phone, he and his collaborators had published evidence of a link between the carotenoids and the ARE. "Our study is focused on the mechanism of how carotenoids like lycopene successfully activate this known protective system in our body which produces these enzymes," Dr. Levy explained. The experiments Dr. Levy and his colleagues performed involved exposing human breast cancer and liver cancer cells to several carotenoids (beta-carotene, lycopene, phytoene, and phytofluene; these last three are found in tomatoes). The results showed that, while all of these carotenoids were able to induce the ARE, lycopene's effect was much greater. Other scientists had previously considered the possibility lycopene could help lower cancer risk, but the mechanism for such an effect was unknown. Dr. Levy's team had found new and important evidence of why lycopene is protective." What is new is that we have shown that the lycopenes [sic] and other carotenoids are the most active phytochemicals when it comes to turning on this antioxidant response system," Dr. Levy explained. This is the mechanism which helps prevent cancer."

Attack of the (cancer- killing) tomatoes: lycopene triggers apoptosis

It's said that truth is often stranger than fiction, and even though there actually *was* a low-budget, 1950's-era horror movie made featuring tomatoes that kill people, no one would have ever imagined that tomatoes might kill *cancer* cells too. Yet this conclusion is supported by research on two of the most common malignancies: prostate and breast cancer. Harvard University Nutrition and Epidemiology Professor Dr. Ed Giovannucci reviewed epidemiological studies that had been published by other scientists, and was one of the first to develop the hypothesis that lycopene may lower cancer risk. He found that 57 out of 72 studies (nearly 80%) concluded that the more lycopene-containing foods people ate, the lower the risk for *several* types of cancer.

Why would tomatoes, out of all other fruits and vegetables, have the power to reduce cancer risk? It's known that tomatoes have both vitamin C and a phytochemical named *quercetin* that is even more powerful an antioxidant than vitamin C, but these may be only part of the reason. A more likely basis for an anti-cancer effect may be concluded from studies done with lycopene both in the laboratory and in men with prostate cancer. These found that lycopene triggers apoptosis through two effects on the IGF-1 axis: IGF-1 levels decrease as the amount of cooked tomatoes we eat increases, while IGF binding proteins increase.

The strongest evidence shows that lycopene is most protective against prostate cancer especially. Significantly lower blood and tissue levels of lycopene, *but not other carotenoids,* have been found in men with prostate cancer. The question about lycopene that remains to be answered is: In studies where tomato-containing foods seemed to lower cancer risk, was it a result of lycopene itself, or was it an effect of lycopene-containing *foods* (i.e., a combined effect of lycopene with the other phytochemicals, vitamins, and minerals found in tomato products)?

Researchers at the University of Illinois at Chicago attempted to answer this question in a study looking at the effect of tomato-containing foods in men with prostate cancer. I called Dr. Phyllis Bowen, the lead investigator in this study, to get some insight into this topic. Dr. Bowen, a Nutrition researcher working in the University's Department of Human Nutrition and Dietetics, made it clear why foods were used in place of lycopene supplements in this study: "As a Nutritionist, I was concerned that the epidemiological studies all pointed to the fact that the protective effect of lycopene was from *foods*, not just certain phytochemicals," she began. "Tomatoes have a number of compounds that could help to reduce cancer risk, including quercetin and other carotenoids, so it could be some synergy between these that account for the anti-cancer effect."

Given the potential anti-cancer synergy between these phytochemicals, why do most studies on lycopene and prostate cancer use lycopene in pill form instead of foods? Dr. Bowen explained: "The problem in testing tomatoes and why everyone uses lycopene capsules is that if you ask for grant money from the National Institutes of Health, they will reject your request if you want to use a food like tomato sauce, because it's not chemically defined – the active phytochemicals and nutrients in it will vary from batch to batch." (Eventually, Dr. Bowen was able to get research funding from tomato products manufacturer Hunt-Wesson instead. However, the use of isolated phytochemicals is clearly counterproductive for scientific research on diet and cancer prevention, because, as Dr. Bowen suggested, people don't eat pills, they eat food.)

Dr. Bowen's study involved thirty-two men who were given foods to eat for three weeks prior to surgical removal of the prostate. These meals consisted of pasta, cheese, and meat, and contained six ounces of the 'active ingredient' (tomato sauce). Results were striking: PSA levels decreased significantly, indicating a possible reduction in prostate cancer progression. "We were surprised that PSA had dropped in that short amount of time, but not sure of our results, because we had no control group," Dr. Bowen noted. The tomato sauce-containing meals also significantly lowered a marker of DNA damage (8OHdG) in both prostate tissue and white blood cells. Perhaps most important was the finding that apoptosis was higher in the surgically removed prostate tissue. Dr. Bowen suggests that the optimistic overall results be considered cautiously, because some men in the study had massive apoptosis, some moderate, and some hardly any at all, "So not everyone was getting the benefit of the tomato-containing foods," she concluded. [*Note:* One could speculate that the reason a better response wasn't obtained might be that the meat and cheese in these entrees are sources of animal protein, saturated fat, and cholesterol, which can raise IGF-1 and contribute to inflammation, both of which can contribute to cancer growth. This type of study badly needs to be repeated, perhaps by giving volunteers tomato sauce with macaroni alone, instead].

Dr. Bowen's research seemed to indicate that tomatoes, not necessarily lycopene itself, have anti-cancer effects in the human body. Scientists at Ohio State University (OSU) came to the same conclusion, after giving prostate cancer-afflicted animals either plain lycopene or tomato powder. Although the lycopene supplement appeared to only slightly reduce prostate cancer death, mortality in tomato-fed animals dropped by 18% compared to animals given neither lycopene nor tomatoes. "Our study does not say that lycopene is useless," said study co-author Dr. Steven K. Clinton during an interview. "Instead it suggests that if we want the health benefits of tomatoes, we should eat tomatoes or tomato products and not rely on lycopene supplements alone." Dr. Bowen's comments were in agreement. "We do *not* know that lycopene is the active, cancer risk-reducing compound," she emphasized. "The best evidence so far are the studies that show a lower risk in people who eat tomato products often. People can get amounts of lycopene that are considered protective as part of their five or more servings of fruits and vegetables per day, even counting ketchup and tomato sauce as a serving," she concluded.

Researchers who are asked to make recommendations regarding diet tend to err on the side of foods, not supplements, as Dr. Giovannucci did when we corresponded by E-mail. When I asked his opinion of more recent studies that concluded lycopene doesn't have a cancer-preventing effect, he didn't object. "I'm not 100% convinced of lycopene either," he opined. "I think the evidence is better worded: 'some item(s) in tomatoes may be beneficial for cancer prevention' because, from the epidemiologic evidence, almost all of the lycopene is from tomatoes. There is no observational or randomized evidence to date that a lycopene *supplement* is beneficial - it may be, but there is no real evidence that addresses this," he concluded.

Getting your lycopene from fruits and vegetables instead of supplements may net you additional benefits, in the form of other carotenoids with anti-cancer effects. One of these is beta-carotene, a vitamin A-like carotenoid found in broccoli, mango, and carrots; another called lutein is found in corn and green vegetables. Both these carotenoids triggered apoptosis and reversed the ability of cancer cells to resist chemotherapy in experimental studies, although evidence of doing so in humans is lacking so far.

What if you're a guy who's skeptical about his risk for prostate cancer? If you plan on living into age 50 and beyond, there are other reasons to be concerned about prostate health. One of these is *benign prostatic hypertrophy* (BPH), a swelling of the prostate that is very common, developing in roughly half of men in this age group. Prescription drugs can deal with BPH symptoms effectively, but if you consider that BPH is also linked with a greater risk for prostate cancer, you may come to the conclusion that you need to do more for prostate health than visit the Doctor and the pharmacy. There are two strategies you can use. Since growth factors (including IGF-1) and foods that increase IGF-1 (mainly animal proteins like red meat, poultry, and eggs) have been linked to development of BPH, strategy number 1 should be to cut back on animal protein. Strategy number 2 should be to add lycopene-containing foods, since this can help prevent BPH symptoms (like prostate enlargement) from getting worse.

BPH symptoms can also wake you up (and your partner as well, unless she is a very sound sleeper) several times each night, which is more than just an inconvenience. Loss of sleep itself is a risk factor for cancer, particularly breast cancer in women. So even if you're not concerned about your own risk for prostate cancer, you should be concerned about an impact of sleep deprivation on your partner's cancer risk.

People at risk for malignancies other than cancer of the prostate also may benefit from a higher lycopene intake. Lycopene lowered IGF-1 in women with a family history of breast cancer, and this may be critical for this sub-group of patients. According to the Endogenous Hormones and Breast Cancer Collaborative Group (a group of 55 researchers from 18 countries) higher levels of IGF-1 have been strongly implicated in breast cancer. Pooling the results of 17 studies involving nearly 5,000 women with breast cancer, these researchers concluded that women with the highest IGF-1 levels had a nearly 40% greater risk for estrogen-receptor-positive tumors, compared with women with the lowest levels. Lycopene supplements reduced IGF-1 by 25% in one clinical study of patients with colon cancer, while another study in persons at very high risk for colon cancer found that lycopene significantly increased the IGF binding proteins that render IGF-1 unable to exert a pro-growth effect on cancer cells.

Lycopene's ability to reduce cancer risk doesn't stop after helping with detoxification, triggering apoptosis, or inhibiting growth factors. This phytochemical also puts a damper on the ability of cancer cells to replicate themselves, as I found out when talking with Dr. Yoav Sharoni, a colleague of Dr. Levy.

Carotenoids: putting a nail in the cell cycle's tire

Dr. Sharoni, a Professor in the Department of Clinical Biochemistry at Ben-Gurion University, is one member of a team that discovered how lycopene activates the antioxidant response element (ARE), a virtual fire department called into action to extinguish the damage caused by free radicals. He and his co-workers also demonstrated lycopene's inhibition of cell cycle progression in breast, lung, and endometrial cancer cells. "Lycopene reduced cyclin D and CDKs," Dr. Sharoni stated during our conversation. "It also prevented the progression from the G1 to the S phase, which is critical. Without the S phase, there's no DNA synthesis and no cancer."

According to Dr. Sharoni, a combination of food carotenoids works against the cell cycle more effectively together than lycopene or beta-carotene alone. "We observed a synergistic effect between the tomato carotenoids on cell cycle inhibition," he continued. "You can't say that lycopene alone or beta carotene inhibits cell cycle proteins. It's a combination of these with the phytoene, phytofluene, and other tomato compounds that have these effects. That's why people should eat foods and not rely on supplements to prevent cancer," he concluded.

Work by Dr. Sharoni and his colleagues have continued to reveal a benefit of carotenoids, at least under experimental conditions. These studies found that in breast cancer cells, several carotenoids prevented estrogen from having pro-growth effects. Nevertheless, they allowed a pro-growth effect of estrogen on normal (bone) cells. If this kind of selective action is revealed to occur in the human body as well, it will point the way even more clearly towards healthy eating for cancer prevention.

Do scientists know for sure that carotenoids keep cancer cells from multiplying in the human body, as well as in the laboratory? The simple answer is they don't, so any recommendations to include carotenoid-containing foods for cancer prevention has to rely on studies of human populations, and there are no shortage of these. Several studies have documented a connection between higher carotenoid intakes and lower risk for breast cancer. However, women who have already dealt with breast cancer may also benefit. In a study which included more than 1500 women in remission for breast cancer, those who had the highest blood levels of carotenoids had a more than a 40% lower risk for recurrence, compared with women with the lowest blood levels. In the aptly named EPIC study (European Prospective Investigation Into Cancer) which included more than a half million women and men, certain carotenoids were inversely associated with gastric cancer risk. (An inverse association means the more you are exposed to a certain condition or substance, the lower your risk). Although carotenoids haven't been associated with a reduced risk for other major cancers (lung, colon and rectum), high intakes of fruits and vegetables have. This may indicate that other nutrients found in fruits and vegetables are more critical to the prevention of these cancers than carotenoids are. Alternately, the carotenoids could simply be playing more limited, behind-the-scenes roles, including that of contributing to a healthy immune system, which also helps to lower your cancer risk.

Immunity thrives on carotenoids

While most parents aren't experts in nutrition or immunology (and even less are familiar with *nutritional* aspects of immunity) most share at least a vague suspicion that eating well is important for our defense against germs. To stress the importance of fruits and vegetables for strong immunity, we often insist that our children eat ("C'mon - just one more bite!") some of these every day. Parents should keep fighting the good fight: studies on carotenoids and immunity show your efforts aren't in vain. The difference to your immune system between eating generous amounts of fruits and vegetables and eating few may be the difference between a terminal diagnosis and staying cancer free.

Some of the first evidence that carotenoids support immunity in humans came from studies showing that high-dose beta-carotene increases the activity of *natural killer* (NK) cells, a kind of immune cell that specifically destroys cancer cells. Fascinatingly, beta-carotene seems to *selectively* improve natural killer cell activity in those who need it most. If you're well nourished and healthy, you may not need the immune-boosting benefits from beta-carotene. However, your elderly parents and/or grandparents, who *are* at greater risk for immune suppression and cancer, can't afford the luxury of passing on carotenoid-containing foods.

Carotenoids support immunity in other ways besides affecting NK cells. Beta-carotene and lutein (a carotenoid found in especially high amounts in green leafy vegetables) activate immune cells called *macrophages* that both destroy bacteria and work with T-cells to enhance your immunity. Carotenoids also protect immune cells from 'friendly fire,' the harmful free radicals they release against their targets. And, through creation of *gap junctions* (channels connecting cells that allow information exchange), carotenoids aid communication between immune cells, a necessity for them to launch a coordinated attack.

Even if you don't have time or desire to cook vegetables, you may still be able to get the amount of carotenoids your immune system needs to work. Mixed vegetable juices significantly increase T-cell function, so you can drink your way to better immunity if you don't eat your veggies at home or work. And while your immune system is enjoying a boost, there's another benefit to this more enlightened way of eating. You'll enjoy the gift of an even lower cancer risk, as your DNA becomes more able to protect and repair itself.

Carotenoids protect your DNA and the skin you're in

One of the benefits of eating a diet higher in minimally processed plant foods and less animal products is that we take in less, and excrete more, DNA-damaging toxins. This is critical for reducing your cancer risk, because DNA damage is an underlying cause of mutations that lead to cancer. Most people think that cancers are events that occur by accident, later in life, and without our ability to interfere with the process. If they only knew that gradual DNA damage that occurs throughout life was a major cause of cancer, they might work harder to protect their DNA.

As with most human functions, our DNA integrity is governed to some degree by what we get from our parents. There are unfortunately no easy ways to screen a population of millions for the inherited ability to prevent or repair DNA damage. Yet because it's known that people who have a poorer ability to repair DNA damage are at greater cancer risk, developing such a test would clearly be of preventive value. In the meanwhile, hedging our best by doing what we can to protect our DNA seems like a good idea. We can work towards this goal by keeping our diets focused on avoiding toxin-containing foods and eating more foods that contain DNA-protecting antioxidants and any nutrients known to help with DNA repair.

There are more specific reasons to work towards these goals than just a general focus on keeping your DNA intact. Taking the case of breast cancer, several studies have found that women with breast cancer have a greater degree of DNA damage in breast tissue specifically, when compared with women without breast cancer. These women may get more benefit from eating DNA-protecting phytochemicals than women at lower breast cancer risk. Similar findings of greater DNA damage have been found in patients at risk for gastric cancer and in smokers, while both a greater extent of DNA damage *and* defective DNA repair is common in patients with head and neck cancers. Some of this influence is genetic, but DNA damage may proceed at a faster rate over a period of many years if you eat an antioxidant-poor (i.e., Western) diet.

Dr. Andrew Collins, a Professor of Nutrition at Norway's University of Oslo, was one of the first scientists to investigate the role of natural compounds on DNA damage and repair. When I spoke with him, he'd recently published evidence of the DNA-protective effects of kiwifruit. "We set out to detect if levels of vitamin C in the blood that were increased by eating kiwifruit translated into a decrease in DNA damage," he began. "When we took lymphocytes [white blood cells] out of the blood of people who'd been eating kiwifruit for a couple of weeks and compared these with persons not eating kiwi, we found a significantly lower amount of DNA damage."

Many phytochemicals have been found capable of reducing DNA damage, which is a testament to the antioxidant power that healthy foods possess. However, relatively few have the ability to impact DNA directly; carotenoids appear to be an exception. In the first study ever to show a protective effect of diet on genetic damage, German investigators gave healthy humans tomato juice, a source of lycopene, and carrot juice, a source of alpha-carotene for several weeks. Although the study included only twenty-three men, the researchers found evidence of both a reduction in DNA damage and an increase in DNA repair.

A follow-up to this study was conducted by the UK's Institute of Food Research, in which Professor Sian Astley and her co-workers exposed human volunteers to one of three treatments. These included alpha- and beta-carotene in pill form, cooked carrots, or a placebo, followed by a comparison of the effects of these treatments on DNA damage and repair. The results indicated a benefit of foods over supplements. Although the beta-carotene supplement more rapidly reduced DNA damage than did the cooked carrots, only those volunteers eating the vegetables showed both a reduction in DNA damage *and* evidence of DNA repair.

More recently, Dr. Collins and his colleagues found evidence from laboratory studies that another carotenoid called cryptoxanthin, found in pumpkin, papaya, red bell pepper, orange juice, tangerines, corn and peas, protects against DNA damage and enhances DNA repair. Interestingly, cryptoxanthin showed these effects at concentrations close to those found in human blood. Studies have also linked higher intakes of this carotenoid with a lower risk for cancers of the breast, kidney, oral cavity, stomach, and ovaries.

With skin cancer on the rise, we may also soon be looking to carotenoids for protection against the DNA damage caused by ultraviolet (UV) light. Dermatologists know that reddening of skin (erythema) is associated with the sort of DNA damage in skin that can increase the risk for skin cancer. A number of laboratory and human studies have demonstrated that the carotenoids increased the amount of time skin could handle being exposed to the sun before erythema developed. Interestingly, carotenoids shared these properties with a number of other phytochemicals, including those present in green tea and cocoa. At the cellular level, scientists found not only less DNA damage and enhanced DNA repair; they also found dramatic reductions in certain enzymes (metalloproteinases) cancer cells use to invade and metastasize.

In spite of these results, the results of large population studies have revealed that taking beta-carotene *pills* is associated with a *greater* risk for skin cancer. In studies where people took antioxidant supplements (a combination of vitamins C, E, beta-carotene, and the minerals selenium and zinc), *skin cancer risk was found to actually decline after stopping daily supplementation.* If this creates confusion about whether or not antioxidants cause or reduce the risk for skin cancer, keep two ideas in mind. First, cumulative DNA damage to your skin over a lifetime of sun exposure is what contributes to your risk for skin cancer, so preventive strategies like a healthy diet must be applied for decades. Second, humans were never exposed to high doses of antioxidant supplements during our evolution. Our genes can't be fooled into thinking that being exposed to high doses of certain nutrients over a small amount of time provides the same benefits as a lifetime of exposure to the lower amounts found in foods.

Beta-carotene: The right 'A' for differentiation to occur

As I discussed in Chapter One, differentiation is a process by which an unspecialized (stem) cell becomes a specialized cell that belongs to your skin, heart, lung, immune system, or other tissue. This process is faulty in cancer cells, and an important goal of cancer therapy involves getting these cancer stem cells to differentiate back to a normal type of cell. Phytochemicals have shown some promise for impacting differentiation in ways that can help lower cancer risk.

A diet rich in vitamin A may be our best bet for getting cancer cells to take this path to differentiation. Laboratory studies have shown that this vitamin triggers differentiation in both normal and malignant cells. I spoke with Dr. Kedar Prasad, Director of Colorado University's Center for Vitamins and Cancer Research, about the benefits of getting vitamin A from beta-carotene, rather than preformed vitamin A, found in high-fat animal foods such as egg yolk and milk. "Beta-carotene affects differentiation in isolated cells apart from its conversion to vitamin A," he explained. "It works by increasing the expression of *connexin* genes. These genes are expressed at low levels in tumor cells, and their increase is a sign cells have become differentiated," he continued. "Connexin genes also increase production of what are called 'gap junction' proteins between cells. Gap junction proteins hold normal cells together, and don't let them divide in an uncontrolled manner," he concluded.

How good is the evidence that carotenoids lower cancer risk?

The evidence from studies in human populations is, unfortunately, not as straightforward as the mechanisms might suggest. Taking breast cancer as an example, a nearly equal number of studies show that carotenoids do and don't lower risk. Further studies have come to a wide variety of conclusions about carotenoids and breast cancer risk. These have determined that only some women with certain sub-types of breast cancer may get a benefit from higher carotenoid intakes. The ways that women differ from each other, including being current/former smokers vs. never-smokers; having dense vs. less dense breasts; having tumors that are hormone-responsive and/or more aggressive vs. those that are not; the type of study done (retrospective vs. prospective, case-control vs. observational); and whether the data come from estimated food intakes vs. blood levels of carotenoids, among others, have all been considered when judging the evidence for an effect of carotenoids on cancer risk. Although the controversy continues, one of the most recent publications had good news about a benefit of fruits, vegetables, carotenoids and breast cancer risk. Researchers from the Imperial College London's School of Public Health looked at all the prospective studies on both fruit and vegetable intake and on the estimated dietary intake vs. blood levels of carotenoids with regard to breast cancer risk. They concluded that women who eat the most fruits and vegetables have a roughly 11% lower risk than those eating the least, and that only blood levels of beta-carotene were truly associated with lower breast cancer risk.

The data get even more interesting when researchers look specifically at high-risk groups. In one of these situations, breast density, a strong risk factor for breast cancer, was viewed in regard to how it might be affected by diet. Comparing roughly 600 women with breast cancer and 600 without, the investigators found that only the high-risk, high breast density group was affected by the amount of carotenoids in their blood. Specifically, those with the highest blood levels had a 40%-50% lower breast cancer risk, compared with the women with the lowest carotenoid levels.

This evidence is helpful, but other kinds of studies have come to different conclusions, so these are clearly not the last word. However, considering the results of some other kinds of studies might be helpful in deciding if eating more carotenoid-containing foods is worth the effort. Studies in women with breast cancer and breast cancer *survivors*, though limited, have revealed that women having higher fruit, vegetable, and carotenoid intakes have either a much lower chance of breast cancer recurrence, or a lower risk of dying from *any* cause.

With respect to other studies, the data haven't supported the ability of carotenoids to lower the risk for colon, rectum, skin, and lung cancers. Several studies with limited amounts of human subjects indicate that eating carotenoid-containing foods may help protect against ovarian, cervical, and uterine cancers, but more studies are needed to confirm this. However, focusing on getting more carotenoids *can* be expected to lower your risk for gastric cancer and cancers of the oral cavity (mouth, tongue, lip, esophagus, and pharynx). In spite of others coming to different conclusions, the World Cancer Research Fund found "substantial and convincing" evidence that lycopene-containing foods *probably* protect against prostate cancer. One of the largest studies ever done on this topic, the 'EPIC' study involving 137,000 men, had an especially interesting outcome. Although carotenoids had no relation to developing *localized* prostate cancer, the risk for *advanced* (metastatic) disease was about 60% lower for men with the highest blood lycopene levels, compared with those with the lowest blood levels. The risk was even lower (65% less) when the amount of blood carotenoids was compared between the highest and lowest groups. This finding is critical, because localized prostate cancer is actually common, and not considered life threatening, in contrast to advanced disease. So it is all the more important that researchers have begun to find that diet makes a difference in whether prostate cancer progresses or remains dormant. In two of these studies, the highest intake of tomato sauce was linked with a 44% lower chance of having a progressive cancer, and adding one serving per day of tomato sauce was linked with experiencing a 50% lower risk for cancer progression.

Getting enough lycopene: a right way and a wrong way?

Adding tomato-based foods to one's diet appears to be good for prostate health. But there may be a right way and a wrong way to get your lycopene, because many foods that have generous amounts of this carotenoid are decidedly *un*healthy.

The evidence is clear that tomato sauce provides both higher amounts and better absorption (because of the added fat helping your gut absorb this fat-soluble nutrient) of lycopene than watermelon, guava, fresh tomatoes, or even tomato juice. However, lycopene-rich foods also include pizza, lasagna and manicotti, and the 'parmigiana' dishes that consist of fried chicken, veal, or eggplant covered with mozzarella cheese. Every one of these is laden with saturated fat, cholesterol, and glycotoxins that are known to promote the type of low-level inflammation associated with greater cancer risk. Toss in some of that aged grated cheese (a rich source of oxidized cholesterol and other pro-inflammatory substances) and you'll pump up the inflammation another notch, while raising your risk for a heart attack. Add to this the animal protein found in both meat and cheese, which raises the cancer-promoting growth factor IGF-1, and you wind up working at cross purposes by eating one food that lowers cancer risk while ingesting several compounds that increase risk. It's also cause to wonder if this type of cuisine was responsible for the results of the few studies that revealed a *higher* risk for breast and prostate cancers in persons with the highest blood lycopene levels, which are contrary to what would be expected from previous research.

Clearly, the safest, *healthiest* way to get your lycopene is putting generous amounts of tomato sauce over macaroni - especially the whole grain types. If you buy or create a sauce with olive oil as an ingredient, chances are you'll increase the anti-cancer benefit, We know this because a systematic review of 19 studies concluded that people in the highest category of olive oil consumption had an almost 60% lower risk for having *any* type of cancer. An even greater anti-cancer benefit could be found by combining the tomatoes and olive oil with beans and garlic, in the traditional Italian dish called *pasta e fagioli*. One other way I've found to maximizing lycopene's benefit is to make your own pizza, using soy cheese, a whole grain pizza crust available at specialty food stores like Trader Joe's or Whole Foods, and some veggies. An increasing number of restaurants that specialize in gourmet pizza also offer these. You can also use a ground beef substitute and soy-based Italian sausage, and make Italian-style foods that are cholesterol-free, low in saturated fat, and high in fiber. These are surprisingly good for mock versions, especially if you load up on fresh garlic, fresh basil, and a homemade tomato sauce with some red wine added. If you should decide to use whole grain noodles in the process, you'll bring the number of cancer-preventing phytochemicals up to near maximum. Creating other meals that are similar in their use of phytochemical-dense foods, and making a habit of doing so at most meals, will help you to enjoy both good food and lower cancer risk at the same time.

CHAPTER FIVE

Crucifers Against Cancer

Although there is without a doubt a certain percentage of people who just don't like vegetables, it would be nearly impossible to find anyone who doesn't agree that they are among the most health-promoting of foods. Nutritionists advise people to not discriminate against any type of vegetable, and to get as wide a variety as possible, in order to increase your chances of getting all the nutrients you need. However, if we had to pick one group of these to eat while stuck on a desert island for life, the evidence suggests that the cruciferous vegetables would make the best choice. These vegetables detoxify carcinogens, ramp up protective antioxidant enzymes and reduce inflammation, help to trigger the self-destruct (apoptosis) pathway in cancer cells, inhibit angiogenesis, keep cancer cells from proliferating, and impact hormone metabolism in ways that help lower your risk for some common cancers. What more could you want from a vegetable?

Detoxification of Carcinogens

The vegetables that comprise the cruciferous vegetable group - including cauliflower, cabbage, Brussels sprouts, turnips, kohlrabi, bok choy, radishes, rapini (broccoli rabe), watercress, wasabi, collards, and the 'crown jewel of nutrition,' broccoli - raise blood levels of certain (Phase II) enzymes responsible for detoxifying potential carcinogens. Many different groups of investigators throughout the world have made valuable contributions to our understanding of the anti-cancer effects of these vegetables. However, the scientist who has done more than anyone else is Dr. Paul Talalay, a Professor of Pharmacology and Director of the Laboratory for Molecular Sciences at Johns Hopkins University School of Medicine. Dr. Talalay was also kind enough to take time out when I asked him to explain the origin of his research on diet and cancer.

During our interview, Dr. Talalay recalled reading research published in 1970 by Lee Wattenberg, a scientist who found that feeding animals a class of phytochemicals called flavones (found in oranges and grapefruit) made it much harder to induce cancer. "We found out that the way these worked was by induction of a whole series of Phase II enzymes," he began. "We wanted to see if inducing these enzymes with certain foods could turn out to be a viable strategy that could protect human beings against cancer. What we did was to go out to a supermarket and bring a lot of different foods, including a lot of vegetables, back to the lab. Then we extracted a number of their active compounds and looked for the ones that had the highest quantities of Phase II inducers. This led in 1992 to the discovery that cruciferous vegetables were higher in content of inducers of the phase II response."

One year later, Dr. Talalay found an ally in Jed Fahey, a plant physiologist with a Doctoral degree in human nutrition and a Masters' Degree in Botany. Together, they established a laboratory designed to study plants for their ability to prevent cancer, and continued their work into the active phytochemicals in crucifers that fight cancer. "We then asked what might be responsible for up-regulating the genes that induce Phase II enzymes," he continued. "This led us to a compound named *sulforaphane*, one that was first identified in 1948. We found it especially concentrated in broccoli, and we were eventually able to show it blocked tumor formation."

Sulforaphane belongs to a group known as *isothiocyanates* (ITC's). The distinctive taste of ITC's becomes apparent when we eat wasabi, horseradish, and mustard. And if you're OK with eating uncooked broccoli and cauliflower, so much the better; the ITC's are actually better absorbed raw than when cooked. This difference may explain why scientists found a lower risk for bladder cancer, even in heavy smokers, in people who ate these vegetables raw three times each month, compared to people eating these least often. No protective effect was seen for eating these cooked, possibly because cooking reduces or destroy ITC's.

Importantly, Dr. Talalay's work didn't just focus on the ability of Phase II enzymes to get rid of carcinogens. It's widely believed that cancer is largely the result of genetic changes coming from the toxic effects of chemically unstable compounds and damaging forms of oxygen. His team found evidence that Phase 2 enzyme inducers also increase antioxidant enzymes that quench free radicals that damage DNA. "These enzymes are the principal protective mechanisms of all cells - not only against chemical agents but against *all* oxidants," Dr. Talalay explained.

In spite of the tremendous importance of finding how crucifers help with detoxification, the scientific literature is conflicted on whether or not eating more of these vegetables reduces cancer risk. Tentatively, scientists have concluded that the degree to which eating these veggies is protective depends in part on your genes. More specifically, it will depend on the interactions between the active ingredients in the vegetables, the frequency with which you eat these, and your inherited genetic variation of the Phase II detoxification enzymes, known as polymorphisms (literally, 'many forms').

The often-confusing aspects of this kind of research include the fact that people inherit many different forms of the detoxification enzymes, not simply a copy that works and one that does not. It gets even more complicated when we consider that having a higher activity of detoxification enzymes may not be an advantage if the chemical compound being removed from circulation is a phytochemical with anti-cancer effects. And the literature is in no means in complete agreement on exactly which polymorphisms raise or lower risk in relation to diet. There are just too many variables and too many genetic sub-types that have to be considered before conclusions can be drawn. Even so, there are several other mechanisms by which cruciferous vegetables reduce cancer risk, so eating more of these can only do you good.

Cruciferous vegetables and apoptosis

Apoptosis, the crucial process of self-destruction that's missing in cancer cells, may be restored by diet, and the evidence suggests that eating more cruciferous vegetables can help. Part of their anti-cancer activity is thought to derive from chemical breakdown products of their digestion. These include (but are certainly not limited to) the phytochemicals sulforaphane, indole-3-carbinol, diindolylmethane (DIM), and PEITC (see below). However, new phytochemicals in crucifers are still being discovered (one of the more recent was designated 'erucin'). It will probably be a long time before there comes an end to the discovery of the total number of these that account for all the anti-cancer effects, which are probably synergistic in nature as well.

Broccoli illustrates this concept perfectly. In addition to the several sulfur compounds that are known to oppose cancer growth, it contains flavonoids with potent antioxidant effects, including *quercetin* (also found in onions, tea, apples, pears, and wine) and *kaempferol* (found in green leafy vegetables, raisins, honey, strawberries, among other foods). The benefit of these was demonstrated in an interesting offshoot of the Polyp Prevention Trial, which examined the effectiveness of diet on the recurrence of pre-cancerous colon lesions, or *adenomas*. People eating more foods containing these flavonoids appeared to have a sharply lower risk (roughly 75% less, in fact) for disease recurrence. Two other studies have found associations between higher kaempferol intakes and reductions in the risk for pancreatic cancer. Studies of such associations are not uncommon. However, when a study includes a huge number of people, other researchers sit up and take notice. The first of these (the 'Multiethnic Cohort Study') included over 180,000 volunteers, while the other (a sub-group of the Alpha-tocopherol, beta-carotene Cancer Prevention Study) included 27,000 male smokers. High kaempferol intake was also associated with a 40% lower risk for a sub-type of ovarian cancer in the Nurses Health Study, which included over 66,000 women. A further list of the vitamins and mineral in broccoli would be illuminating but unnecessary. The point is, foods are often exceedingly complex in their make-up, and their anti-cancer benefits are often over-determined, as well as underestimated.

With regard to apoptosis, crucifers accomplish this critical step by decreasing anti-apoptotic proteins and increasing pro-apoptotic proteins. The phytochemical diindoylmethane (DIM) also causes apoptosis by reducing the activity of NFκB, a master regulation of inflammation that is considered necessary for survival by cancer cells. However, by far the most interesting process is one that has been labeled 'intracellular catastrophe.' This occurs through the generation of a massive number of free radicals that destroy their targets with various, toxic forms of oxygen ('prooxidants'). This is fascinating, because many phytochemicals in vegetables are thought to be *anti*oxidants. Just as fascinating is the evidence that these effects occur selectively on cancer cells, not normal ones, making them an ideal form of chemoprevention.

Another way that cruciferous vegetables affect apoptosis is through changing the kind of hormones our bodies create. Estrogen is one of these hormones, and the more women are exposed to it, the greater their risk for breast and other reproductive cancers. Two reasons for the connection between estrogen and female cancers include its' well-known pro-growth effects, and an ability to shut down apoptosis. The reverse is true as well: blocking access to estrogen causes cancer cells to commit apoptosis. Phytochemicals in cruciferous vegetables have an ability to keep estrogen from being changed in the body to a form that may be cancer causing, although this is still controversial (see below). Even so, these vegetables are good sources of dietary fiber, which is more firmly linked to colorectal cancer prevention. We may conclude from this that it's likely you'll get multiple layers of protection from eating these vegetables, even if one of these effects doesn't pan out.

I spoke with Dr. Shivendra Singh, a Professor at the University of Pittsburgh's Department of Pharmacology and Chemical Biology, about work he and his colleagues published involving another phytochemical (phenethyl isothiocyanate, PEITC) in cruciferous vegetables. "We were interested in seeing if the low amounts that could be found in blood were able to cause apoptosis," he began. "We found that in prostate cancer cells exposed for extended periods of time to PEITC, we did in fact see apoptosis occurring."

Like DIM, PEITC affects apoptosis by increasing proteins with pro-apoptotic effects and by decreasing proteins that have *anti*-apoptotic effects. In animals that Dr. Singh's group studied, feeding PEITC significantly retarded the growth of prostate cancer cells these mice had been injected with. Dr. Singh's group also documented that sulforaphane could trigger apoptosis in several types of cancer cells, as well as animals afflicted with prostate cancer. What are the chances that these phytochemicals could do the same in humans? Although he stresses the need for further research, Dr. Singh had a tentative answer. "After being in this field, I'm convinced that if you can regularly consume certain vegetables, for example, like having some broccoli every day, you *will* get the phytochemicals that provide anti-cancer benefits," he opined.

After we had this conversation, a number of epidemiological studies gave additional weight to the possibility of reducing prostate cancer risk through consuming more crucifers. The Prostate, Lung, Colorectal and Ovarian Cancer Screening Trial, which involved over 29,000 men followed for over four years, found an association between the highest intake of cruciferous vegetables and a 40% lower risk for aggressive prostate cancer. In a German cohort of the European Prospective Investigation Into Cancer (EPIC) study that involved over 11,000 men followed up over more than nine years, the highest intake of glucosinolates (the parent compound of many anti-cancer chemicals found in cruciferous vegetables) was associated with a greater than 30% lower risk for prostate cancer.

Cruciferous vegetables and risk for hormone-related cancers

As far as hormone-related cancers go, lowering your risk is possible, but would require changes in your diet that lower the amount of available hormone, prevent hormones from binding to their targets (receptors), and cut down on production of more active forms of hormones. Phyto-chemicals in cruciferous vegetables may be able to affect the latter two processes. "We know that there are a lot of biologically active ingredients in plant foods that can either interfere with the actions of hormone-metabolizing enzymes, or stimulate their synthesis," commented Dr. Cheryl Rock, a Professor of Family and Preventive Medicine at the University of California at San Diego. "For example, they might stimulate the breakdown of hormones including estrogen, or alter the pathway so that not the most *potent* hormone is created," she concluded.

Dr. Rock is referring to studies that revealed estrogen has a greater ability to increase cancer risk (specifically, by damaging DNA) *after* it gets converted to a form called a 'catechol estrogen quinone'. Women with breast cancer make more of this type of estrogen than women without breast cancer do, particularly if they eat diets high in fat and low in fiber. Interestingly, this conversion process is reduced when women eat more broccoli, cauliflower, cabbage, and Brussels sprouts. This may explain why certain studies have suggested that breast cancer risk increases in women who eat the lowest amounts of cruciferous vegetables.

Inhibition of cancer cell proliferation and inflammation with cruciferous vegetables

In addition to reducing the risk for hormone-related cancers, people who eat more cruciferous vegetables appear to have a lower risk for cancers of the colon and lung. One of the keys to these benefits is sulforaphane, a phytochemical with impressive cell cycle-inhibiting effects in lab studies. These include increasing both the tumor suppressor p53 and cell cycle-restraining CDKIs, while inhibiting cyclin D1, CDKs, and the G1 to S progression phase.

   Under laboratory conditions, phytochemicals in cruciferous vegetables also reduce inflammation. Chronic, low-level inflammation drives cancer growth, so we should probably add 'anti-inflammatory' to our list of reasons to eat these vegetables. Inflammation also is a critical underlying factor in cardiovascular disease, diabetes, osteoporosis, arthritis, dementia, and in fact most other diseases. So far, there's evidence that crucifers protect against the two 'biggies' (cardiovascular disease and cancer), and data on the others may be forthcoming.

Chapter Six:

Spice it Up: Add Flavor, Subtract Cancer Risk

No matter how high a food product scores on anyone's list of cancer-fighting potential, one thing is for sure: you won't get people to eat it if it doesn't taste good. Taste has consistently been found to be the number one consideration when people choose what to eat, ranking miles above other concerns such as price, health value, convenience, or other factors.

The palatability of foods is also important to consider if you are trying to lose weight. And make no mistake: keeping excess weight off is *not* an option if you're looking to avoid cancer. Being obese (not just somewhat overweight) raises your risk for some of the most common cancers, including colorectal cancer, breast cancer, and endometrial cancer, in addition to less common types such as esophageal, pancreatic, thyroid, kidney, and gallbladder cancers.

Dieters have to deal several times each day with the option of choosing tastier, weight-gain promoting foods, or the (sometimes) blander-but-better-for you alternative. If the only two choices are eating foods that taste good but cause weight gain, or a cuisine that keeps you trim but just doesn't cut the (flavored) mustard, you're in trouble. There has to be a third option, consisting of foods that are both flavorful *and* low enough in calories to keep the weight off.

Flavoring foods with herbs, spices, and other seasonings may be the perfect way to accomplish this. And according to several groups of cancer researchers, it's also turned out to be one of the best ways to lower cancer risk, and possibly even improve cancer treatment. So far, the best examples science offers in this category includes curcumin (found in turmeric and curry powder) and garlic. In this chapter, I'll review some of the amazing things these can do to help reduce your cancer risk, if you're willing to eat these on a regular basis. Since most readers are likely to be more familiar with using garlic than curry, let's start there.

Detoxifying properties of garlic

Detoxification of cancer-causing carcinogens ultimately involves jettisoning these from the body. However, another step in the prevention of harm from carcinogens involves keeping inert pro-carcinogens from being 'activated' to fully armed chemical poisons. As it turns out, phytochemicals in garlic have the ability to do *both* jobs.

Although detox enzymes are found throughout the body, they are concentrated in the liver, which is considered a type of 'clearinghouse' for all the chemicals, both natural and foreign, that pass through the bloodstream. But taking tissue samples to analyze a person's detoxification abilities isn't easy (think of someone doing a liver biopsy on you with a needle the length of an oil dipstick). While taking skin samples is likely to net more volunteers than a more invasive sample request would, it's easy to understand why most studies on diet and detoxification are done with small animals.

Researchers working in the U.K. approached this problem through a particularly innovative approach. They decided to test the ability of garlic to prevent carcinogen activation by giving volunteers a muscle-relaxant drug (CZX) along with a liquid concentrate (yecch) of a garlic phytochemical called diallyl sulfide (DAS), and by measuring the ratio between the drug's breakdown product and levels of un-metabolized CZX. Results confirmed that the garlic extract put a kink in the Phase I enzymes, and increased the ratio of un-metabolized to metabolized drug.

At the same time they prevents Phase I carcinogen activation, garlic phytochemicals also increase the activity of Phase II detoxification enzymes. In fact, they are so effective for this purpose that garlic oil is traditionally used in treating liver diseases in some countries. Garlic is also able to restore the levels of certain detoxification enzymes (GPx) in alcohol-addicted individuals. Heavy drinking is known to increase your risk for several cancers, and it can take many years for people to stop alcohol abuse. Garlic might therefore represent an opportunity to lower cancer risk in these patients while they are fighting for sobriety.

By itself, an effect on detoxification only partly explains why garlic appears to lower cancer risk. There are several other mechanisms at work here, but studies in humans are needed before recommendations can be made to the public. So it should be comforting for those of you who enjoy garlic-laden foods to know the findings of a Japanese study, in which a significantly smaller size and number of colon adenomas (a pre-cancerous lesion) were found in humans who had taken garlic extract for 12 months, compared with patients who got a placebo. This also dovetails nicely with studies in human populations, which for the most part have revealed garlic's ability (along with other *Allium* family vegetables like onions, scallions, chives, and leeks) to lower the risk for gastric cancers. And although the degree of risk reduction has been estimated as small as 10%, it's a relatively large payoff considering the small amount you have to eat to obtain it, which is a fraction of an ounce each day. There's a bonus, however; in fact, more than one, if you're willing to eat garlic more often. First, there are some large and some smaller studies indicating frequent garlic consumption may help lower the risk for certain hormone-related cancers. And in spite of the Food and Drug Administration's (FDA) assertions that there is "…no credible evidence to support a relation between garlic intake and a reduced risk of gastric, breast, lung, or endometrial cancer" [and] "Very limited evidence [to support] a relation between garlic consumption and reduced risk of colon, prostate, esophageal, larynx, oral, ovary, or renal cell cancers," the FDA's conclusions were drawn with respect to food labeling – meaning, not necessarily applicable to people eating garlic over a period of many years.

The evidence from other studies, as I'll discuss below, argues against FDA's conclusion. Some of these involve specific phytochemicals found in garlic, as opposed to whole garlic intake. In one of these studies, one garlic compound (S-allylmercaptocysteine, SAMC) was able, under experimental conditions, to increase the effectiveness of a chemotherapeutic drug for a particular form of prostate cancer from which few patients survive. This kind of research has been increasing over the past few years, as the ingredients thought to be *the* active principle in foods are isolated and used in a drug-like fashion.

Garlic triggers apoptosis in cancer cells

"In several parts of China where people eat larger amounts of garlic, they seemed to be protected against certain cancers," pointed out Dr. I. Bernard Weinstein, a professor of genetics and development and public health at Columbia University, during a conversation we had about his research on garlic. Prior to his death, Dr. Weinstein and his colleagues isolated a number of garlic phytochemicals (sulfur-containing, or *thiol* compounds) with anti-cancer effects. One of these is SAMC, a phytochemical produced when we digest garlic. SAMC disrupts the ability of cancer cells to create the internal support structure (microtubules) they need to maintain shape, divide, and survive. As a result, an internal wrecking ball that consisting of a protein-munching enzyme called a *caspase* is activated, and apoptosis results. Other phytochemicals in garlic, including *allicin* and *ajoene*, also trigger caspases and apoptosis in both animal and human cancer cells. Ajoene works by reducing *bcl-2*, a protein that opposes apoptosis and shields cancer cells from the effects of chemotherapeutic drugs. Laboratory studies showed that ajoene dramatically increases the pro-apoptosis effect of two commonly used chemotherapy agents. Importantly, ajoene causes apoptosis in human leukemia cells *without* damaging healthy white blood cells. Finding chemicals that selectively cause apoptosis in cancer cells is rare. Yet these are exactly the kind of 'targeted' agents that are desired by the drug discovery research community, because too many other cancer-killing compounds kill the patient's healthy cells too.

Can eating garlic regularly decrease the risk for cancer in humans? I also interviewed Dr. Singh in order to shed some light on this question. "Our lab is working on cancer prevention by nutritional agents, including garlic-derived chemicals like diallyl sulfides," Dr. Singh began. "The chemical that seems to be the most potent one, at least in prostate cancer cells, is called diallyl trisulfide, or DATS, which is quite effective at inducing apoptosis." When asked if eating garlic could achieve blood levels of DATS that might lower cancer risk, Dr. Singh suggested that animal studies might provide the answer. "Some work with another garlic compound called SAC shows that levels attainable in blood did cause apoptosis, so we think that we may be able to get similar results with DATS. We're doing studies in animals now to see if this is the case."

Dr. Singh's group found that, like ajoene, DATS has effects on apoptosis through bcl-2. "DATS not only reduces the levels of bcl-2, but also changes it in other ways too," Dr. Singh explained. One of these changes involves adding phosphorus to bcl-2. "We're working now to show that when this happens, bcl-2 loses its ability to bind and inactivate proteins that would normally trigger apoptosis. As a result, caspases are activated that trigger apoptosis."

Dr. Singh also noted that DATS blocks the ability of certain cancer cells to proliferate. "We also have evidence that besides causing apoptosis, DATS causes something called 'mitochondrial catastrophe' in cancer cells," added Dr. Singh. Mitochondrial catastrophe is a process that, according to Dr. Singh, is not well defined. However, what *is* known is that it involves the creation of incomplete DNA, along with the formation of cells that are temporarily alive, but can't reproduce.

Is it likely that garlic supplements can provide similar benefits for cancer prevention? "I think it's really premature to make a comparison between the effects of isolated phytochemicals and whole foods," Dr. Singh cautioned. "There may be additive or synergistic effects of multiple chemicals involved. We won't know if these are helpful unless very carefully designed studies are done comparing foods with supplements."

Garlic, immunity, and cancer risk

Data that first revealed garlic's ability to kill cancer cells dates back to the late 1950's, and may be where people got the widely-assumed idea that garlic is a 'natural antibiotic' of sorts. Interestingly, garlic works in a remarkably similar way to a vaccine used specifically for the treatment of certain cancers. This vaccine (Bacillus Calmette-Guerin, BCG for short) is an immune system booster that is used in the United Kingdom to prevent children from getting tuberculosis. Like BCG, garlic increases the immune system's natural killer cell activity, triggers T-cell growth and activity, and increase release of cytokines (interleukins, interferon, and tumor necrosis factor, TNF) that amplify your immune response to certain cancers in their early stages.

The immune-supporting benefits of garlic may have practical, real-life applications, including an ability to prevent suppression of the immune system by chemotherapy. One way this may occur is through providing sulfur-containing compounds. These help prevent depletion of the important antioxidant glutathione, which plays key roles in fueling the immune system and producing tumor-killing cytokines like TNF.

Where the rubber meets the road

Does evidence from studies of human subjects with cancer or pre-cancerous conditions reveal that garlic is preventive? Before I provide you with an answer, keep a few things in mind. Most cancers are deadly, and develop over a long period of time as a result of a buildup of damaging mutations. To expect a single food to significantly impact cancer risk is unrealistic, if not foolish. It's more than enough to ask if a *combination* of foods, as part of a life-long dietary pattern, can reduce cancer risk. If one food alone seems to have such a powerful, drug-like effect, it would be nothing short of amazing. Yet the results of two clinical trials in humans come close to this.

Feeding human subjects whole garlic resulted in boosting the ability of their natural killer (NK) cells to kill tumor cells by 40%-60%, when compared with people not given garlic. In patients with colorectal pre-cancerous lesions (adenomas), taking higher amounts of aged garlic extract resulted in a significant decrease in the appearance of new adenomas and suppressed the growth of existing ones, compared to people given lower doses. While these studies do not reveal a chemotherapeutic effect of garlic in patients with an existing cancer, they obviously reveal a chemopreventive effect that may lower the risk for developing future malignancies.

One of a number of interesting trends in research on natural compounds and cancer includes combining the effect of two or more agents to see how much greater the effect may be, when compared with one alone. Because garlic is often used in cooking in the same dishes as curry powder is used, there may be a synergistic effect of the two on cancer growth. This is a tempting hypothesis; for now, let's turn to the data on curcumin (an anti-cancer phytochemical found in curry spice) to see how it can help lower cancer risk.

Curcumin reduces cancer risk by lowering inflammation

Curcumin, as well as garlic, suppresses inflammation by decreasing activity of the same COX-2 enzyme that aspirin and similar drugs called NSAIDs (ibuprofen, naproxen sodium, celecoxib) do. The importance of this is the connection it has with data showing that chronic, low-level inflammation has a key role in increasing cancer risk. The studies on this topic have yielded important findings on the relationships between inflammation, anti-inflammatory strategies, and cancer risk. One of the first important published findings came from Ohio State University researchers, who looked at 91 epidemiological studies on the use of NSAIDs and cancer risk. They found a significant decline in the risk with daily intake of NSAIDs for the four major types of cancer (colon, breast, lung, and prostate cancer). Reductions in risk ranged from 36%-63%, with additional significant risk reductions found for esophageal (73%), stomach (62%), and ovarian cancers of 47% to 73%. Keep in mind, these results were from observational studies, and are not thought to be as 'real-life' as controlled clinical studies are. However, one of the latest and most convincing studies summarized the results of 51 randomized, controlled trials of aspirin and cancer prevention. University of Oxford researchers who reviewed these trials concluded that people who regularly take aspirin have a roughly 25% lower risk for cancer incidence and mortality. Overall, the data are clear that drugs that suppress inflammation lower cancer risk, because inflammation is a key process in cancer growth. As I mentioned earlier, inflammation favors angiogenesis and decreases apoptosis, and involves the release from immune cells of growth factors and cytokines that promote cancer growth.

Given the strong body of data that NSAIDs decrease cancer risk, why is it that more people aren't advised by their physicians to take aspirin or ibuprofen every day? One answer is that there is a *very* strong chance that if you do so, you'll wind up in the hospital with a perforated bleeding ulcer. And although this happens in only between 1–2% of users, somewhere between 3,200 and 16,500 deaths per year are caused by NSAIDs in the United States alone. Obviously, no physician wants to risk harming a patient, even if it means lowering his or her cancer risk. So using herbs and spices to reduce COX-2-activated inflammation is not only a good way to lower cancer risk, it's smarter because it doesn't involve an increased risk for a bleeding ulcer or death.

The research on herbs and spices in cancer prevention, aside from garlic and curcumin, is in its infancy. John Milner, a scientist working for the National Cancer Institute who specializes in the connections between nutrition and cancer, summarized the state of the science recently. The data have revealed anti-cancer effects – at least, in the laboratory – for practically every herb and spice you'll find in your kitchen cabinet. Allspice, basil caraway, cardamom, cinnamon, clove, coriander, cumin, dill, ginger, rosemary, saffron and thyme are biologically active against cancer growth in various ways, although none have been found to act therapeutically (yet). It will probably be several more years before the research on these has advanced enough to determine how potent they truly are. However, that shouldn't keep you from doing your own experiment, while enhancing the taste of your meals in the process.

Chapter 7

A Grape Way to Fight Cancer?

The 'French paradox' refers to the observation that people living in France have far less cardiovascular disease than people in many other developed nations, in spite of their high cholesterol diets. The French differ from Americans in many ways, including diet and activity levels; however, much research on the French paradox has focused on one specific phyto-chemical in one particular beverage: the resveratrol in red wine.

When it comes to *heart* disease, the idea of drinking wine makes sense. Regardless of the type, alcohol raises your 'good' HDL cholesterol, and has a 'thinning' effect on the blood, lowering the tendency of your blood to clot. As a result, having 1 or 2 drinks each day cuts the risk for heart attack and stroke, when compared with being a teetotaler. There's a good chance that your Doctor knows this, and if you ask her, I can summarize in advance the advice you'll receive. You'll be told that, if you drink at all, you should limit your consumption to 1 or 2 drinks each day. You may also be told that if you don't already drink, you shouldn't start. Why? The answer involves your cancer risk, among other potential problems.

When it comes to cancer, don't expect the same encouraging advice to drink moderately that you may get with heart disease. This is because your Doctor also knows that in most studies, with few exceptions, heavier alcohol use is linked with greater cancer risk, particularly for breast cancer. The exceptions to these studies are those that have shown associations between moderate wine drinking and a lower risk for prostate cancer, lung cancer, ovarian cancer, and lymphoma. And not all types of wine have the same association with cancer risk. In a study where alcohol intake was examined in relation to breast density (a risk factor for breast cancer), drinking *white* wine showed up in association with greater risk, while drinking red wine was *inversely* associated with breast density. And a study of alcohol intake and risk for skin cancer involving more than 108,000 people found that alcohol intake increased skin cancer risk, except for red wine, the intake of which was protective (but strangely, only in women).

Dr. Andrew Joe, a scientist with the Herbert Irving Comprehensive Cancer Center at Columbia University, gave his opinion of these studies during a discussion we had about his work on resveratrol and apoptosis. "The data on the anti-cancer effects of resveratrol come mainly from laboratory experiments and population studies," he began. "In some populations where wine is consumed daily and moderately, studies show a lower risk for cancer. We're not talking about large consumption. These individuals are not drinking alcohol every day, which could actually increase the risk of certain cancers, like breast cancer," he continued.

How does it work?

Resveratrol is a phytochemical found in abundance in two beverages: red wine and de-alcoholized red wine. Purple grapes, grape products, and peanuts and raisins also have resveratrol, but far less than red wine. Hundreds of laboratory studies have revealed that resveratrol has a variety of anti-cancer effects. These include acting as an antioxidant, triggering apoptosis, inhibiting angiogenesis and inflammation, preventing carcinogen activation, and even possibly anti-hormone effects.

Resveratrol triggers apoptosis in cancer cells

Dr. Joe explained some of the science behind resveratrol's anticancer effects. "When we looked at proteins involved in cell growth and apoptosis, we found some were affected by resveratrol," he noted. Dr. Fazlul Sarkar, a cancer researcher and Professor at the Wayne State University School of Medicine, explained further, noting that resveratrol's ability to reduce inflammation knocks out several proteins that oppose apoptosis. As a result, resveratrol reduced the size, development, and average number of breast tumors in animals. Importantly, cancer metastasis to the lung was inhibited in these animals, while apoptosis increased.

The question that still needs to be answered is, Can we attain resveratrol levels in blood and tissues high enough to cause apoptosis by consuming resveratrol-containing foods and drinking red wine? Most scientist are skeptical; Dr. Joe cautioned that what goes on in the lab may not be occurring in the human body. However, Dr. Nihal Ahmad, an Asst Professor in the Department of Dermatology at the University of Wisconsin's Comprehensive Cancer Center, was more optimistic. Dr. Ahmad's group studied the effects of resveratrol on survivin, an anti- apoptosis factor found in many cancers. Suppressing survivin is important because doing so results in an increase in sensitivity to drugs that cause apoptosis. "This is just my opinion," stated Dr. Ahmad. "But the amounts needed to produce effects on cancer risk should be achievable in humans with moderate consumption of red wine."

Effects on hormones

One of the most well known ways that drinking alcohol is thought to raise the risk for certain (breast) cancers is by preventing the clearing of estrogen from the blood. Because estrogen acts as a growth factor for breast cancer cells, it's one of the most well researched potential causes of breast cancer, with total lifetime exposure most important in determining risk. In general, women are warned to avoid alcohol totally to keep breast cancer risk low. The problem with this advice is that most women are at higher risk for heart attack and stroke than for breast cancer, and moderate alcohol intake helps lower the risk for both these major killers.

Most research on resveratrol indicates that women may be able to have the best of both worlds. Resveratrol exerts a critical effect on estrogen, that of inhibiting the enzyme aromatase that converts androgens to estrogen. In studies done on isolated breast cancer cells, this effect caused breast cell growth to slow down, and eliminated pre-cancerous and cancerous changes. Resveratrol also inhibited the growth of endometrial cancer cells, while ovarian cancer cells were killed outright by its application. But don't assume that women are the only beneficiaries of this compound; men at risk for prostate cancer might also benefit from resveratrol. Lab studies found this phytochemical suppresses a hormone (androgen) receptor that plays a key role in the development of prostate cancer. Impressive stuff, you might say; and the data become somewhat more impressive when we consider that these effects have also been found in laboratory animals being treated for cancer.

Is there evidence that it works in humans?

Do the effects of resveratrol seen in the laboratory and in animals translate to protection against cancer in humans? To be able to come to any conclusions, we have to weigh the types of evidence that exist. These fall into several categories: lab studies, population studies, and human clinical trials. We've already seen that lab studies are in favor of resveratrol; in fact, it's considered one of the most potent anti-cancer agents ever discovered. Population studies are mixed, with some revealing that *moderate* consumption of red wine is associated with lower risk for a number of cancers. Yet there are just as many studies, if not more, that don't indicate drinking red wine lowers cancer risk. In between these studies, there is a suspicion on the part of many investigators that if red wine and resveratrol have anti-cancer effects, it's because wine is part of a Mediterranean diet. The fruits, vegetables, olive oil, legumes, and whole grain breads in this dietary pattern contain a staggering number of anti-cancer phytochemicals, in addition to relatively high (relative to a Western diet, that is) amounts of protective vitamins and minerals. The Mediterranean diet is however very low in red meat and higher in fish, which may also help lower cancer risk. Put these all together, and you begin to wonder if the focus should be on a single phytochemical in one beverage, or on getting more people to eat a diet that combines healthy foods, such as the Mediterranean diet.

Unfortunately, scientific investigations don't work this way. Single ingredients are the main focus of most researchers, who use their knowledge to extract these active compounds and attempt to prove their worth by giving large doses to willing subjects. In the few studies done this way, resveratrol has been impressive. A study of resveratrol's effect on detoxification enzymes found an increase in certain Phase II detoxification enzymes, but *only* in persons who had low levels to begin with. This implies that these people would experience a greater anti-cancer benefit than people with normal levels of these enzymes. (These data aren't ready for prime time, but could be used eventually if gene profiling were done along with prescribed approaches to cancer prevention involving diet). An inhibition of drug metabolism was also found, implying that resveratrol lowered the activity of Phase I detoxification enzymes. While this could be bad news for anyone taking a wide variety of medications, resveratrol's ability to put a kink in certain Phase I enzymes might lower a woman's ability to make the most active form of estrogen (estradiol), thereby reducing one factor among many in breast cancer risk. We might conclude for the time being that while low amounts of resveratrol might help lower cancer risk, high (i.e., supplementary) amounts might be bad for people who regularly take medicines for pain, blood thinning, and to lower blood sugar and cholesterol, among others.

I interviewed Dr. Andreas Gescher, a Professor of Biochemical Toxicology at the UK's University of Leicester, regarding resveratrol and apoptosis. In a recent study he was involved in, scientists from the National Cancer Institute (NCI) and the University of Michigan Medical School (UMMS) gave human volunteers large doses of resveratrol, ranging from 0.5 to 5 grams per day for roughly one month. Their goal was to find out if, as it had turned out in animal studies, resveratrol could lower IGF-1 and affect its availability by increasing the amount of IGF binding proteins (IGFBP-3). The critical nature of this study was based on evidence in human populations showing that high IGF-1 and low IGFBP-3 levels are related to the risk for cancers of the breast, prostate, lung, colon, and rectum.

The combined results from all groups revealed that resveratrol reduced IGF-1 significantly, although it also lowered IGFBP-3 (possibly because less IGF-1 means less binding protein is needed). The researchers stressed the need to repeat this study, for obvious reasons. If the results pan out as accurate, it could mean that an important step could be taken to lower cancer risk in persons with higher-than-normal IGF-1 levels. It might also mean that one way to oppose the rise in IGF-1 caused by animal protein is by eating and drinking resveratrol-containing foods with the same meal.

More impressive results of resveratrol have recently been found in cancer patients. In another joint venture between UK's University of Leicester, the NCI and UMMS, high doses of resveratrol resulted in a 5% decrease in the proliferation of tumor cells in 20 persons with confirmed colorectal cancer. You might think at first that a 5% reduction is hardly worth the effort. However, other studies with high doses of phytochemicals, including curcumin and the catechins in green tea, for example, also found reductions in cancer proliferation. Almost certainly, one of the next steps investigators take will be to combine these to see how much better cancers can be controlled.

In a second clinical trial, high doses of highly absorbable (micronized) resveratrol were again given to patients with colorectal cancer; this time however, it was with a group of patients with metastatic cancer. This study, rather than being funded by the NCI or UMMS, was funded in part by the drug company GlaxoSmithKline. This time, results were more impressive: a marker of apoptosis was increased by nearly 40% in the malignant liver tissue. These results imply a potential role for resveratrol alongside chemotherapy or radiation, possibly by allowing lower doses of both to be used (to avoid toxicity) while still allowing the elimination of cancer cells.

To drink or not to drink?

Drinking red wine isn't for everyone; many people prefer white wine or beer, and many avoid alcohol for reasons related to health or religious beliefs. But if you don't have a seriously good reason to avoid drinking, you should actually consider it a preventive health strategy, much like exercise or taking a baby aspirin once each day. Although cancer prevention should be a major consideration in your lifestyle, you should also consider that, according to the best research available, small amounts of alcohol – as little as 1 serving per day – can lower your risk for most major killers of Americans. Having 1-2 alcohol-containing drinks each day lowers your cardiovascular death risk by about 25%, compared with not drinking. If you choose to drink less often, you can still get a cardiovascular benefit, and you'll cut your risk for the most common type of (ischemic) stroke by roughly 20%. Consuming roughly 1.5 drinks per day has even turned out to protect against adult-onset diabetes by about 40% in women and 13% in men. Interestingly, diabetes is associated with greater risk for many cancers, so it seems strange that drinking alcohol – an excess of which is linked with *higher* risk for many cancers – can actually lower cancer risk through diabetes prevention. If we consider the risk for cardiovascular disease, kidney disease, eye disease, nerve disease and amputations linked with diabetes, it begins to seem as if *everyone* over the age of 21 should be drinking nearly daily and in moderation. It should however be remembered that amounts higher than 2 drinks per day has the opposite effect, increasing the risk for a multitude of diseases.

But why red wine? The data are very clear that *any* kind of alcohol provides these benefits, whether it's red wine or moonshine. There are still some reasons that drinking red wine is of greater benefit than other kinds of alcohol. One of these is an effect on blood pressure. While alcohol *per se* tends to raise blood pressure, there's evidence that the phytochemicals in red wine actually lower it. Perhaps this is because red wine is a source of antioxidants, which is another unique benefit of this kind of alcoholic beverage. (Most types of alcohol are not only devoid of antioxidants, but also have a 'pro-oxidant' effect: i.e., they cause production of the free radicals that use up part of your body's supply of antioxidants).

How do I get resveratrol if I don't drink?

There are sources of resveratrol other than red wine, including peanuts, grapes, and soy foods for example; it's just that red wine has larger amounts. The two ways you can get large amounts of resveratrol without drinking are to use red wine frequently in cooking (add to spaghetti sauce, for example) or to drink Itadori tea, a traditional herbal remedy for heart disease and strokes used in Japan and China. The second requires that you find the raw material to make Itadori tea, which comes from Japanese knotweed. This is known to be a very invasive species, so if you plant it, make sure you avoid sharing it with your neighbors, unless you want to be stuck with a hefty landscaping bill. De-alcoholized red wine is available, and boiled peanuts will net you more resveratrol than raw ones.

Chapter Eight:

The Grain Gain: How Whole Grains Fight Cancer

If I asked you to guess where the majority of cancer-fighting antioxidant phytochemicals are found, you would probably say that fruits and vegetables contain the lion's share. Surprisingly, whole grains are even richer sources. The combined presence of the antioxidants and fiber in whole grains may explain why people eating diets high in whole wheat, oats, rye and other whole grains have significantly lower risks for stomach cancer, colon cancer, and cancers of the oral cavity (lip, tongue, and esophagus). Whole grain eaters also weigh less, an important key for cancer prevention, than people who eat refined grain (i.e., white flour) products.

Why is there such a difference in cancer risk between eating whole grains compared to refined grains? Dr. David Jacobs, an Epidemiologist from the University of Minnesota's School of Public Health, provided one answer when we discussed his research. Over the past 15 years, Dr. Jacobs has almost single-handedly championed studies of the health benefit of whole grains in disease prevention. He's worked on a number of landmark studies (The Iowa Women's Health Study and the Cancer Prevention Study II Nutrition Cohort). These involved tens of thousands of individuals, in efforts to track how whole grains and other foods impact the risk for cancer, diabetes, cardiovascular disease, and other chronic health problems. He's also written more extensively than just about anyone else regarding the synergistic effect of protective nutrients found in plant foods. I didn't have to go further than a conversation with Dr. Jacobs to understand why whole grains are preferred to refined ones for cancer-prevention.

"Refined grains eliminate anything that has biological activity," Dr. Jacobs began. "So any nutrient or phytochemical you can think of that is protective, you've eliminated 85%-90% by refining the grain. In general, I think it's extremely likely that synergy between these substances is the most important thing that happens in what you eat."

The phytochemicals in whole grains and legumes inhibit cancer growth by several mechanisms. Apart from the benefit of phytochemicals, whole grains also provide fiber, which, although it never leaves the gut, exerts powerful anticancer effects outside the GI tract regardless. Fiber binds hormones; lowers the availability of growth factors (IGF-1, insulin) that turn the cell cycle; and binds and lowers cholesterol, which also causes cell cycle arrest.

Whole grain and legume fiber provide two additional benefits. First, they contribute *inositol hexaphosphate* (IP6, also known as phytate or phytic acid), a unique phytochemical with numerous anti-cancer effects. Second, dietary fiber's effect in the colon causes gut bacteria to ferment the fiber, thereby releasing *butyric acid,* which steps up levels of cell cycle-restraining CDKIs in colon cancer cells, while allowing proliferation of normal colon cells. I'll provide more specific details below on how these work against cancer, starting with IP6.

Inositol hexaphosphate: a 'hex' with magical effects?

Dr. Rajesh Agarwal was kind enough to speak with me in order to detail some of the anti-cancer benefits of IP6. I also received some help from Dr. Ivana Vucenik, an Associate Professor at the University of Maryland Medical School who has done groundbreaking work on IP6 and cancer prevention. Both mentioned that IP6 has antioxidant effects, prevents progression of the cell cycle, enhances both immunity and the anticancer effect of chemotherapy, and helps control cancer metastases. In addition to all these mechanisms, IP6 also increases differentiation of cancer cells. Impressive effects, when we consider that we can achieve these life-saving effects by doing simple things like eating bran flakes instead of Choco-Puffs and tossing some chickpeas into your salad. "IP6 is found in high amounts in cereals, legumes, and whole grains, especially the bran," noted Dr. Vucenik. "However, in addition to plant cells, IP6 is also found in almost all human and animal cells, in substantial amounts."

Many of the pioneering experiments on the anticancer effect of IP6, including the induction of differentiation of malignant cells, was performed on IP6 by Dr. Vucenik and her colleague, Dr. AbulKalam Shamsuddin, at the University of Maryland Medical School's Department of Medical and Research Technology. Together, they showed that the breakdown products of IP6 (inositol phosphates) might be responsible for the effect of IP6 on tumor differentiation. "Induction of terminal differentiation and decreasing the elevated rate of cell proliferation are two basic mechanisms for the anti-cancer effect of IP6," Dr. Vucenik confirmed. "We've seen this in leukemia cell lines, in breast cancer, colon cancer, prostate cancer, all the ones that are so affected by diet and nutrition. We've also seen these effects in liver and sarcoma cancer cells," she continued. "In almost every kind of malignant cell, we saw that IP6 was actually able to *reverse* malignancy. It's also selective, not affecting or harming normal cells, and is cyto*static* [inhibiting growth or duplication], not cyto*toxic* like drugs."

Dr. Vucenik also voiced the opinion that IP6 might work more effectively when combined with other phytochemicals. "There has been a study where IP6 was given with green tea, and there was synergism," she confirmed. "We also showed that there's a synergism between IP6 and standard chemotherapy that's important in cancer treatment."

Studies on IP6 confirms the benefits of whole grain in our diets, and underscore the recent suggestion by the Dietary Guidelines for Americans Committee to eat three or more servings of whole grain foods each day, in place of refined grains. "I think we should be eating all of our grain products from whole grains, not refined ones," Dr. Vucenik suggested, "but we can't make recommendations for this based on what we know so far." (Although this is true, it is also a fact that no one is actually recommending we eat refined grains, or suggesting whole grains are harmful for prevention of any kind of disease, gluten fanatics aside).

IP6 appears to work a large part of its anti-cancer magic by preventing cancer proliferation. According to Dr. Agarwal, IP6 opposes the cancer cell cycle by decreasing the CDKs that push the cell cycle forward, increasing cell cycle-restraining CDKIs, and lowering cyclin D1 protein levels. It restores the function of tumor suppressor genes that have been compromised, one of which is the Rb (short for retinoblastoma) protein. Cancer cells that are exposed to IP6 are basically forced to either 'join the rank or walk the plank'- they either differentiate into normal, non-cancerous cells or undergo apoptosis.

Interestingly, IP6 interferes with cancer cell division without affecting healthy cells. "This is one of the most interesting things about IP6," Dr. Agarwal began. "In prostate cancer cells, IP6 selectively induces CDK inhibitors *without* affecting non-cancerous prostate tissue. When we took out those genes, IP6 didn't have the same inhibiting effect on the cell cycle, indicating that this phytochemical was working through the tumor suppressor proteins to get that response," he continued. Dr. Agarwal also indicated a potential role for IP6-rich diets in cancer treatment. "In animals where we've used IP6, we see a strong response in terms of preventing and treating different cancers," he began. "That suggests that the amount that works in cell cultures is absolutely achievable in the body, without any toxicity."

One additional benefit of IP6 includes the ability to trigger differentiation (discussed below). These benefits aside, it shouldn't be forgotten that whole grains and legumes have other antioxidant phytochemicals, vitamins, and minerals that can help lower cancer risk. One of these, the mineral magnesium, also inhibits cell cycle progression in certain types of cancer cells, and may also inhibit cancer growth through an anti-inflammatory effect.

The many benefits of a high-fiber diet

For many years, eating a high-fiber diet has been thought of as a possible way to protect against colon cancer. One of the more positive studies found a greater than 40% reduction in colorectal cancer risk among 52,000 women and men eating the highest amount of dietary fiber, compared with those eating the least. Another large study found that people at the greatest risk for colorectal cancer were those eating very low amounts of fiber (less than 10 grams per day). The benefits of eating more fiber-containing foods on colorectal cancer risk is generally thought to be due to fiber's ability to dilute and bind bile acids, so that they don't exert toxic effects on the colon wall. The jury is still out on whether everyone gets the same cancer-lowering benefit from eating large amounts of fiber, or if a threshold exists above or below which there's a point of diminishing return. However, there's evidence that suggests the benefits of fiber are derived in part from a substance that your gut produces from fiber, rather than fiber itself. The effect of this compound on differentiation may be the reason.

Digestion of fiber produces what are called 'short-chain fatty acids' (SCFAs). These are made in the colon when bacteria that live there break down dietary fiber. SCFAs are thought to act as a fuel for the cells lining the colon, helping them to absorb nutrients. One of these SCFAs (*butyrate*) plays a number of roles in colon health. Butyrate stimulates detoxification enzymes (glutathione-S-transferases); reduces inflammation; and inhibits a key enzyme, histone deacetylase, which results in a decreased ability of cancer cells to proliferate. "Butyrate is important not only as a source of energy for colon cells, but also to regulate genes that control differentiation, cell division, and cell death," explained Soraya Shirazi-Beechey, a Professor of Molecular Physiology and Biochemistry at the University of Liverpool. Dr. Beechey's group discovered an important reason, involving butyrate metabolism, why higher fiber intakes don't always appear to lower the risk for colorectal cancer.

Dr. Beechey and her co-workers found that the mere presence of butyrate doesn't have a protective effect; it needs a certain protein to get into colon cells. However, in certain kinds of colon cancer cells, a defect exists in getting butyrate into these cells. The result: no entry, no gene regulation, and no differentiation. In other words, the lack of being able to transport butyrate into colon cells may explain why, at least in some people, high-fiber diets may not protect against this cancer.

"When we knocked out the expression of this protein in our studies, we find that some of these butyrate-related genes become dysregulated," explained Dr. Beechey. "What we have shown in patients with colon cancer is that very early on during the development of this disease, there's a down-regulation of this protein," explained Dr. Beechey. "In people who don't benefit from fiber in terms of reduced colorectal cancer risk, there's hardly any of this protein, so butyrate can't get into the cells to regulate these genes." Part of this defect, explained Dr. Beechey, may be genetic in origin. "There are different forms of this butyrate transport protein we call MCT-1," she continued. "These aren't reflective of any functional defect, but it causes the signaling pathway that gets butyrate into cells to become defective, sort of like the way that people with Type 2 diabetes have a problem getting insulin to make glucose transporters that bring sugar into cells."

Butyrate may have applications in other cancers too. Researchers have been testing a form of butyrate (sodium phenylbutyrate) in patients with prostate cancer and certain blood cancers, with some success. However, experimental data indicate that butyrate doesn't work as well by itself as it does in the presence of other fiber-derived SCFAs. In some of these studies, SCFAs produced from a dietary fiber mixture inhibited the growth of colon cancer cells even more than mixtures of short-chain fatty acids with or without butyrate alone. In fact, the whole fiber mixture boosted butyrate's anti-cancer effects. "We know that when fiber or resistant starch is fermented in the colon, we get other SCFA's, and these are equally important as regulators of butyrate absorption and gene expression," commented Dr. Beechey.

Another class of phytochemicals that can help trigger differentiation are called *sterols*. These are found in oils, seeds and nuts, cereals, and legumes. (If the word 'sterol' sounds familiar, it's because sterols form part of *chole*sterol. Plant sterols keep us from absorbing cholesterol, and are now used by millions of Americans in the form of certain brands of margarine, to lower blood cholesterol). The most common plant sterol is called beta-sitosterol. At the cellular level, beta-sitosterol activates a process called the *sphingomyelin cycle*. Through this cycle, sphingomyelin breaks down, and *ceramide* is produced, which causes differentiation. The diagram below helps to better illustrate this process:

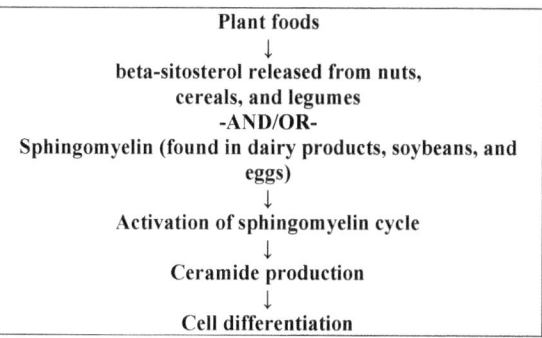

It's very likely that other mechanisms by which whole grains protect against cancer will be found. However, the evidence is already clear enough to exchange your meat for legumes, whole grains, and nuts and seeds.

References

Introduction: A New Approach to Understanding and Preventing Cancer

1. Wang C, Miller SM, Egleston BL, Hay JL, Weinberg DS. Beliefs about the causes of breast and colorectal cancer among women in the general population. Cancer Causes Control. 2010 Jan;21(1):99-107.
2. National Breast Cancer Coalition Survey Reveals That Heightened Breast Cancer Awareness Has Insufficient Impact on Knowledge. Accessed 12-4-2007 at: http://www.medicalnewstoday.com/articles/84216.php
3. World Cancer Research Fund / American Institute for Cancer Research. Policy and Action for Cancer Prevention. Food, Nutrition, and Physical Activity: a Global Perspective. Washington DC: AICR, 2009

Chapter One: Next Stop, Cancerville: why everyone you know is on the same train

Aggarwal BB, Takada Y, Oommen OV. From chemoprevention to chemotherapy: common targets and common goals. Expert Opin Investig Drugs. 2004 Oct;13(10):1327-38.

Ahn J, Gammon MD, Santella RM et al. Effects of glutathione S-transferase A1 (GSTA1) genotype and potential modifiers on breast cancer risk. Carcinogenesis. 2006 Sep;27(9):1876-82.

Aljada A, Ghanim H, Mohanty P, Syed T, Bandyopadhyay A, Dandona P. Glucose intake induces an increase in activator protein 1 and early growth response 1 binding activities, in the expression of tissue factor and matrix metalloproteinase in mononuclear cells, and in plasma tissue factor and matrix metalloproteinase concentrations. Am J Clin Nutr. 2004 Jul;80(1):51-7.

Allen NE, Appleby PN, Davey GK, Key TJ. Hormones and diet: low insulin-like growth factor-I but normal bioavailable androgens in vegan men. Br J Cancer. 2000 Jul;83(1):95-7.

Allen NE, Key TJ, Appleby PN et al. Animal foods, protein, calcium and prostate cancer risk: the European Prospective Investigation into Cancer and Nutrition. Br J Cancer. 2008 May 6;98(9):1574-81.

American Cancer Society. Cancer Facts & Figures 2008. Atlanta: American Cancer Society; 2008.

Ames BN, Gold LS. Dietary carcinogens, environmental pollution, and cancer: some misconceptions. Med Oncol Tumor Pharmacother. 1990;7(2-3):69-85.

Annenberg/CPB. Interview with Robert Weinberg on cell biology and cancer. Expert Interview Transcript series. Available at: http://www.learner.org/channel/courses/biology/units/cancer/experts/weinberg.html.

Ardies CM, Dees C. Xenoestrogens significantly enhance risk for breast cancer during growth and adolescence. Med Hypotheses. 1998 Jun;50(6):457-64.

Astley SB, Elliott RM. How strong is the evidence that lycopene supplementation can modify biomarkers of oxidative damage and DNA repair in human lymphocytes? J Nutr. 2005 Aug;135(8):2071S-3S.

Aubertin-Leheudre M, Gorbach S, Woods M, Dwyer JT, Goldin B, Adlercreutz H. Fat/fiber intakes and sex hormones in healthy premenopausal women in USA. J Steroid Biochem Mol Biol. 2008;112(1-3):32-9.

Balkau B, Kahn HS, Courbon D, Eschwège E, Ducimetière P; Paris Prospective Study. Hyperinsulinemia predicts fatal liver cancer but is inversely associated with fatal cancer at some other sites: the Paris Prospective Study. Diabetes Care. 2001 May;24(5):843-9.

Badria FA. Melatonin, and tryptamine in some Egyptian food and medicinal plants. J Med Food. 2002 Fall;5(3):153-7.

Bagga D, Anders KH, Wang HJ, Glaspy JA. Long-chain n-3-to-n-6 polyunsaturated fatty acid ratios in breast adipose tissue from women with and without breast cancer. Nutr Cancer. 2002;42(2):180-5.

Baillargeon J, Rose DP. Obesity, adipokines, and prostate cancer (review). Int J Oncol. 2006 Mar;28(3):737-45.

Barnard ND, Scialli AR, Hurlock D, Bertron P. Diet and sex-hormone binding globulin, dysmenorrhea, and premenstrual symptoms. Obstet Gynecol. 2000 Feb;95(2):245-50.

Barnard RJ. Prostate cancer prevention by nutritional means to alleviate metabolic syndrome. Am J Clin Nutr. 2007 Sep;86(3):s889-93.

Barnard RJ, Aronson WJ. Preclinical models relevant to diet, exercise, and cancer risk. Recent Results Cancer Res. 2005;166:47-61.

Barone J, Hebert JR, Reddy MM. Dietary fat and natural-killer-cell activity. Am J Clin Nutr. 1989 Oct;50(4):861-7.

Bartella V, Cascio S, Fiorio E, Auriemma A, Russo A, Surmacz E. Insulin-dependent leptin expression in breast cancer cells. Cancer Res. 2008 Jun 15;68(12):4919-27.

Bartsch C, Bartsch H. Melatonin in cancer patients and in tumor-bearing animals. Adv Exp Med Biol. 1999;467:247-64.

Bastard JP, Jardel C, Bruckert E et al. Elevated levels of interleukin 6 are reduced in serum and subcutaneous adipose tissue of obese women after weight loss. J Clin Endocrinol Metab 2000 Sep;85(9):3338-42.

Bauer M, Herbarth O, Rudzok S, Schmücking E, Müller A, Aust G, Gräbsch C. Diversity of common alternative splicing variants of human cytochrome P450 1A1 and their association to carcinogenesis. Int J Oncol. 2007; Jul;31(1):211-8.

Bennett FC, Ingram DM. Diet and female sex hormone concentrations: an intervention study for the type of fat consumed. Am J Clin Nutr. 1990 Nov;52(5):808-12.

Bhargava A. Fiber intakes and anthropometric measures are predictors of circulating hormone, triglyceride, and cholesterol concentrations in the women's health trial. J Nutr. 2006 Aug;136(8):2249-54.

Brandt B, Hermann S, Straif K, Tidow N, Buerger H, Chang-Claude J. Modification of breast cancer risk in young women by a polymorphic sequence in the egfr gene. Cancer Res. 2004 Jan 1;64(1):7-12.

Bongartz T, Sutton AJ, Sweeting MJ, Buchan I, Matteson EL, Montori V. Anti-TNF antibody therapy in rheumatoid arthritis and the risk of serious infections and malignancies: systematic review and meta-analysis of rare harmful effects in randomized controlled trials. JAMA. 2006 May 17;295(19):2275-85.

Boynton A, Neuhouser ML, Wener MH et al. Associations between healthy eating patterns and immune function or inflammation in overweight or obese postmenopausal women. Am J Clin Nutr. 2007 Nov;86(5):1445-55.

Britton JA, Khan AE, Rohrmann S et al. Anthropometric characteristics and non-Hodgkin's lymphoma and multiple myeloma risk in the European Prospective Investigation into Cancer and Nutrition (EPIC). Haematologica. 2008 Nov;93(11):1666-77.

Brody JG, Moysich KB, Humblet O, Attfield KR, Beehler GP, Rudel RA. Environmental pollutants and breast cancer: epidemiologic studies. Cancer. 2007 Jun 15;109(12 Suppl):2667-2711.

Carruba G, Granata OM, Pala V et al. A traditional Mediterranean diet decreases endogenous estrogens in healthy postmenopausal women. Nutr Cancer. 2006;56(2):253-9.

Carluccio MA, Siculella L, Ancora MA et al. Olive oil and red wine antioxidant polyphenols inhibit endothelial activation: antiatherogenic properties of Mediterranean diet phytochemicals. Arterioscler Thromb Vasc Biol. 2003 Apr 1;23(4):622-9.

Carmeliet P. Manipulating angiogenesis in medicine. J Intern Med. 2004 May; 255(5):538-61.

Caserta D, Maranghi, serotonin L, Mantovani A, Marci R, Maranghi F, Moscarini M. Impact of endocrine disruptor chemicals in gynecology. Hum Reprod Update. 2008 Jan-Feb;14(1):59-72.

Chalabi N, Delort L, Le Corre L, Satih S, Bignon YJ, Bernard-Gallon D. Gene signature of breast cancer cell lines treated with lycopene. Pharmacogenomics. 2006 Jul;7(5):663-72.

Chan HY, Leung LK. A potential protective mechanism of soya isoflavones against 7,12 dimethylbenz[a] anthracene tumour initiation. Br J Nutr. 2003 Aug;90(2):457-65.

Chang D, Wang F, Zhao YS, Pan HZ. Evaluation of oxidative stress in colorectal cancer patients. Biomed Environ Sci. 2008 Aug;21(4):286-9.

Chen P, Hu P, Xie D, Qin Y, Wang F, Wang H. Meta-analysis of vitamin D, calcium and the prevention of breast cancer. Breast Cancer Res Treat. 2010 Jun;121(2):469-77.

Chen YQ, Edwards IJ, Kridel SJ, Thornburg T, Berquin IM. Dietary fat-gene interactions in cancer. Cancer Metastasis Rev. 2007 Dec;26(3-4):535-51.

Chiu BC, Cerhan JR, Folsom AR, Sellers TA, Kushi LH, Wallace RB, Zheng W, Potter JD. Diet and risk of non-Hodgkin lymphoma in older women. JAMA. 1996 May 1;275(17):1315-21.

Cho E, Spiegelman D, Hunter DJ, Chen WY, Stampfer MJ, Colditz GA, Willett WC. Premenopausal fat intake and risk of breast cancer. J Natl Cancer Inst. 2003 Jul 16;95(14):1079-85.

Chuma M, Hige S, Nakanishi M, Ogawa K, Natsuizaka M, Yamamoto Y, Asaka M. 8-Hydroxy-2'-deoxy-guanosine is a risk factor for development of hepatocellular carcinoma in patients with chronic hepatitis C virus infection. J Gastroenterol Hepatol. 2008 Sep;23(9):1431-6.

Cross AJ, Peters U, Kirsh VA, Andriole GL, Reding D, Hayes RB, Sinha R. A prospective study of meat and meat mutagens and prostate cancer risk. Cancer Res. 2005 Dec 15;65(24):11779-84.

Chan C. Childhood obesity and adverse health effects in Hong Kong. Obes Rev. 2008;9 Suppl 1:87-90.

Chow HH, Hakim IA, Vining DR et al. Modulation of human glutathione s-transferases by polyphenon e intervention. Cancer Epidemiol Biomarkers Prev. 2007 Aug;16(8):1662-6.

Collins AR. Antioxidant intervention as a route to cancer prevention. Eur J Cancer. 2005;41(13):1923-30.

Collins AR, Harrington V, Drew J, Melvin R. Nutritional modulation of DNA repair in a human intervention study. Carcinogenesis. 2003 Mar;24(3):511-5.

Collier AC, Dandge SD, Woodrow JE, Pritsos CA. Differences in DNA-damage in non-smoking men and women exposed to environmental tobacco smoke (ETS). Toxicol Lett. 2005 Jul 28;158(1):10-9.

Cross HS, Kállay E, Lechner D, Gerdenitsch W, Adlercreutz H, Armbrecht HJ. Phytoestrogens and vitamin D metabolism: a new concept for the prevention and therapy of colorectal, prostate, and mammary carcinomas. J Nutr. 2004 May;134(5):1207S-1212S.

Darling JA, Laing AH, Harkness RA. A survey of the steroids in cows' milk. J Endocrinol; 1974: 62:291–297.

Dawson-Hughes B, Harris SS, Rasmussen H, Song L, Dallal GE. Effect of dietary protein supplements on calcium excretion in healthy older men and women. J Clin Endocrinol Metab. 2004 Mar;89(3):1169-73.

Dewell A, Weidner G, Sumner MD et al. Relationship of dietary protein and soy isoflavones to serum IGF-1 and IGF binding proteins in the Prostate Cancer Lifestyle Trial. Nutr Cancer. 2007;58(1):35-42.

Dhawan V, Jain S. Garlic supplementation prevents oxidative DNA damage in essential hypertension. Mol Cell Biochem. 2005 Jul;275(1-2):85-94.

Dorai T, Aggarwal BB. Role of chemopreventive agents in cancer therapy. Cancer Lett. 2004;215:129-40.

Dorgan JF, Judd JT, Longcope C et al. Effects of dietary fat and fiber on plasma and urine androgens and estrogens in men: a controlled feeding study. Am J Clin Nutr. 1996 Dec;64(6):850-5.

Drummond S, Dixon K, Griffin J, De Looy A. Weight loss on an energy-restricted, low-fat, sugar-containing diet in overweight sedentary men. Int J Food Sci Nutr. 2004 Jun;55(4):279-90.

Dumitrescu RG, Cotarla I. Understanding breast cancer risk -- where do we stand in 2005? J Cell Mol Med. 2005 Jan-Mar;9(1):208-21.

Endogenous Hormones, Prostate Cancer Collaborative Group. Endogenous Sex Hormones and Prostate Cancer: A Collaborative Analysis of 18 Prospective Studies. JNCI 2008; 100(3):170-183.

Erba D, Riso P, Bordoni A, Foti P, Biagi PL, Testolin G. Effectiveness of moderate green tea consumption on antioxidative status and plasma lipid profile in humans. J Nutr Biochem. 2005 Mar;16(3):144-9.

Faguet GB. The War on Cancer: An Anatomy of Failure, A Blueprint for the Future. Dordrecht, The Netherlands: Springer, 2005.

Fair AM, Dai Q, Shu XO et al. Energy balance, insulin resistance biomarkers, and breast cancer risk. Cancer Detect Prev. 2007;31(3):214-9.

Fair AM, Montgomery K. Energy balance, physical activity, and cancer risk. Methods Mol Biol. 2009;472:57-88.

Fairfield KM, Hunter DJ, Colditz GA, Fuchs CS, Cramer DW, Speizer FE et al. A prospective study of dietary lactose and ovarian cancer. Int J Cancer. 2004 ;110:271-7.

Fenech M. The Genome Health Clinic and Genome Health Nutrigenomics concepts: diagnosis and nutritional treatment of genome and epigenome damage on an individual basis. Mutagenesis. 2005 Jul;20(4):255-69.

Fenech M. Genome health nutrigenomics and nutrigenetics--diagnosis and nutritional treatment of genome damage on an individual basis. Food Chem Toxicol. 2008 Apr;46(4):1365-70.

Federico A, Morgillo F, Tuccillo C, Ciardiello F, Loguercio C. Chronic inflammation and oxidative stress in human carcinogenesis. Int J Cancer 2007 Dec 1;121(11):2381-6.

Fontana L, Weiss EP, Villareal DT, Klein S, Holloszy JO. Long-term effects of calorie or protein restriction on serum IGF-1 and IGFBP-3 concentration in humans. Aging Cell. 2008 Oct;7(5):681-7.

Food and Nutrition Board/IOM. Dioxins and Dioxin-like Compounds in the Food Supply: Strategies to Decrease Exposure. Washington DC: National Academy of Sciences, 2003.

Flood A, Mai V, Pfeiffer R et al. The effects of a high-fruit and -vegetable, high-fiber, low-fat dietary intervention on serum concentrations of insulin, glucose, IGF-I and IGFBP-3. Eur J Clin Nutr. 2008 Feb;62(2):186-96.

Frattaroli J, Weidner G, Dnistrian AM et al. Clinical events in prostate cancer lifestyle trial: results from two years of follow-up. Urology. 2008 Dec;72(6):1319-23.

Ford ES. Prevalence of the metabolic syndrome defined by the International Diabetes Federation among adults in the U.S. Diabetes Care. 2005 Nov;28(11):2745-9.

Fulgoni VL. Current protein intake in America: analysis of the National Health and Nutrition Examination Survey, 2003-2004. Am J Clin Nutr. 2008 May;87(5):1554S-1557S.

Gallus S, Scotti L, Negri E et al. Artificial sweeteners and cancer risk in a network of case-control studies. Ann Oncol. 2007 Jan;18(1):40-4.

Gann PH, Kazer R, Chatterton R et al. Sequential, randomized trial of a low-fat, high-fiber diet and soy supplementation: effects on circulating IGF-I and its binding proteins in premenopausal women. Int J Cancer. 2005 Aug 20;116(2):297-303.

Gao D, Wei C, Chen L, Huang J, Yang S, Diehl AM. Oxidative DNA damage and DNA repair enzyme expression are inversely related in murine models of fatty liver disease. Am J Physiol Gastrointest Liver Physiol. 2004 Nov;287(5):G1070-7.

Gerl R, Vaux DL. Apoptosis in the development and treatment of cancer. Carcinogenesis. 2005;26(2):263-70.

Ghadirian P, Thouez JP, PetitClerc C. International comparisons of nutrition and mortality from pancreatic cancer. Cancer Detect Prev. 1991;15(5):357-62.

Gilmore TD, Herscovitch M. Inhibitors of NF-kappaB signaling: 785 and counting. Oncogene. 2006 Oct 30;25(51):6887-99.

Giovannucci E, Pollak M, Liu Y, Platz EA, Majeed N, Rimm EB, Willett WC. Nutritional predictors of insulin-like growth factor I and their relationships to cancer in men. Cancer Epidemiol Biomarkers Prev. 2003 Feb;12(2):84-9.

Giovannucci E, Rimm EB, Stampfer MJ, Colditz GA, Ascherio A, Willett WC. Intake of fat, meat, and fiber in relation to risk of colon cancer in men. Cancer Res. 1994 May 1;54(9):2390-7

Goldman R, Shields PG. Food mutagens. J Nutr. 2003 Mar;133 Suppl 3:965S-973S.

Grifantini K. Understanding pathways of calorie restriction: a way to prevent cancer? J Natl Cancer Inst. 2008 May 7;100(9):619-21.

Grubben MJ, Nagengast FM, Katan MB, Peters WH. The glutathione biotransformation system and colorectal cancer risk in humans. Scand J Gastroenterol Suppl. 2001;(234):68-76.

Grundy SM. Metabolic syndrome pandemic. Arterioscler Thromb Vasc Biol. 2008 Apr;28(4):629-36.

Guadagni F, Ferroni P, Palmirotta R, Portarena I, Formica V, Roselli M. Review. TNF/VEGF cross-talk in chronic inflammation-related cancer initiation and progression: an early target in anticancer therapeutic strategy. In Vivo. 2007 Mar-Apr;21(2):147-61.

Guarnieri S, Riso P, Porrini M. Orange juice vs vitamin C: effect on hydrogen peroxide-induced DNA damage in mononuclear blood cells. Br J Nutr. 2007 Apr;97(4):639-43.

Gunter MJ, Hoover DR, Yu H et al. Serum C-peptide, IGFBP-1 and IGFBP-2 and risk of colon and rectal cancers in the European Prospective Investigation into Cancer and Nutrition. Cancer Res. 2008 ;68(1):329-37.

Gunter MJ, Hoover DR, Yu H et al. Insulin, insulin-like growth factor-I, and risk of breast cancer in postmenopausal women. J Natl Cancer Inst. 2009 Jan 7;101(1):48-60.

Gunter MJ, Stolzenberg-Solomon R, Cross AJ et al. A prospective study of serum C-reactive protein and colorectal cancer risk in men. Cancer Res. 2006 Feb 15;66(4):2483-7.

Guyton KZ, Kensler TW, Posner GH. Vitamin D and vitamin D analogs as cancer chemopreventive agents. Nutr Rev. 2003 Jul;61(7):227-38.

Habdous M, Siest G, Herbeth B, Vincent-Viry M, Visvikis S. Glutathione S-transferases genetic polymorphisms and human diseases: overview of epidemiological studies. Ann Biol Clin (Paris). 2004 Jan-Feb;62(1):15-24.

Hallett WH, Murphy WJ. Natural killer cells: biology and clinical use in cancer therapy. Cell Mol Immunol. 2004 Feb;1(1):12-21.

Hammarsten J, Högstedt B. Hyperinsulinaemia: a prospective risk factor for lethal clinical prostate cancer. Eur J Cancer. 2005 Dec;41(18):2887-95

Han J, Hankinson SE, Ranu H, De Vivo I, Hunter DJ. Polymorphisms in DNA double-strand break repair genes and breast cancer risk in the Nurses' Health Study. Carcinogenesis. 2004 Feb;25(2):189-95.

Han J, Hankinson SE, Colditz GA, Hunter DJ. Polymorphisms in DNA double-strand break repair genes and skin cancer risk. Cancer Res. 2004 May 1;64(9):3009-13.

Hankin JH, Rawlings V. Diet and breast cancer: a review. Am J Clin Nutr. 1978 Nov;31(11):2005-16.

Harris JE. Smoke yields of tobacco-specific nitrosamines in relation to FTC tar level and cigarette manufacturer: analysis of the Massachusetts Benchmark Study. Public Health Rep. 2001 Jul Aug;116(4):336-43.

Harvie M, Howell A. Energy balance adiposity and breast cancer - energy restriction strategies for breast cancer prevention. Obes Rev. 2006 Feb;7(1):33-47.

Haydon AM, Macinnis RJ, English DR, Morris H, Giles GG. Physical activity, insulin-like growth factor 1, insulin-like growth factor binding protein 3, and survival from colorectal cancer. Gut. 2006;55(5):689-94.

Heald AH, Cade JE, Cruickshank JK, Anderson S, White A, Gibson JM. The influence of dietary intake on the insulin-like growth factor (IGF) system across three ethnic groups: a population-based study. Public Health Nutr. 2003 Apr;6(2):175-80.

Heald AH, Sharma R, Anderson SG et al. Dietary intake and the insulin-like growth factor system: effects of migration in two related populations in India and Britain with markedly different dietary intake. Public Health Nutr. 2005 Sep;8(6):620-7.

Hebert JR, Barone J, Reddy MM, Backlund JY. Natural killer cell activity in a longitudinal dietary fat intervention trial. Clin Immunol Immunopathol. 1990 Jan;54(1):103-16.

Herman-Giddens ME, Slora EJ, Wasserman RC, Bourdony CJ, Bhapkar MV, Koch GG, Hasemeier CM.

Secondary sexual characteristics and menses in young girls seen in office practice: a study from the Pediatric Research in Office Settings network. Pediatrics. 1997 Apr;99(4):505-12.

Hetts SW. To die or not to die: an overview of apoptosis and its role in disease. JAMA. 1998 Jan 28;279(4):300-7.

Hiipakka RA, Zhang HZ, Dai W, Dai Q, Liao S. Structure-activity relationships for inhibition of human 5alpha-reductases by polyphenols. Biochem Pharmacol. 2002 Mar 15;63(6):1165-76.

Holick CN, Newcomb PA, Trentham-Dietz A et al. Influence of a diet very high in vegetables, fruit, and fiber and low in fat on prognosis following treatment for breast cancer: the Women's Healthy Eating and Living (WHEL) randomized trial. Cancer Epidemiol Biomarkers Prev. 2008 Feb;17(2):379-86.

Holtzclaw WD, Dinkova-Kostova AT, Talalay P. Protection against electrophile and oxidative stress by induction of phase 2 genes: the quest for the elusive sensor that responds to inducers. Adv Enzyme Regul. 2004;44:335-67.

Hoppe C, Mølgaard C, Michaelsen KF. Cow's milk and linear growth in industrialized and developing countries. Annu Rev Nutr. 2006;26:131-73.

Hoppe C, Udam TR, Lauritzen L, Molgaard C, Juul A, Michaelsen KF. Animal protein intake, serum insulin-like growth factor I, and growth in healthy 2.5-y-old Danish children. Am J Clin Nutr. 2004 Aug;80(2):447-52.

Howell WM, Calder PC, Grimble RF. Gene polymorphisms, inflammatory diseases and cancer. Proc Nutr Soc. 2002 Nov;61(4):447-56

Howie BJ, Shultz TD. Dietary and hormonal interrelationships among vegetarian Seventh-Day Adventists and nonvegetarian men. Am J Clin Nutr. 1985 Jul;42(1):127-34.

Hsing AW, Chu LW, Stanczyk FZ. Androgen and prostate cancer: is the hypothesis dead? Cancer Epidemiol Biomarkers Prev. 2008 Oct;17(10):2525-30.

Inadera H. The usefulness of circulating adipokine levels for the assessment of obesity-related health problems. Int J Med Sci. 2008 Aug 29;5(5):248-62.

Ingram DM, Bennett FC, Willcox D, de Klerk N. Effect of low-fat diet on female sex hormone levels. J Natl Cancer Inst. 1987 Dec;79(6):1225-9.

Inoue T, Inoue K, Maeda H, Takayanagi K, Morooka S. Immunological response to oxidized LDL occurs in association with oxidative DNA damage independently of serum LDL concentrations in dyslipidemic patients. Clin Chim Acta. 2001 Mar;305(1-2):115-21.

Ishizuka B, Quigley ME, Yen SS. Pituitary hormone release in response to food ingestion: evidence for neuroendocrine signals from gut to brain. J Clin Endocrinol Metab. 1983 Dec;57(6):1111-6.

Jakobisiak M, Lasek W, Golab J. Natural mechanisms protecting against cancer. Immunol Lett. 2003 Dec 15;90(2-3):103-22.

Jenab M, Riboli E, Cleveland RJ et al. Serum C-peptide, IGFBP-1 and IGFBP-2 and risk of colon and rectal cancer: The European Prospective Investigation into Cancer and Nutrition. Int J Cancer. 2007 Jul 15;121(2):368-76.

Jolliffe CJ, Janssen I. Vascular risks and management of obesity in children and adolescents. Vasc Health Risk Manag. 2006;2(2):171-87.

Joseph MA, Moysich KB, Freudenheim JL et al. Cruciferous vegetables, genetic polymorphisms in glutathione S-transferases M1 and T1, and prostate cancer risk. Nutr Cancer. 2004;50(2):206-13.

Juret P, Couette JE, Mandard AM, Carre A, Delozier T, Brune D, Vernhes JC. Age at menarche as a prognostic factor in human breast cancer. Eur J Cancer. 1976 Sep;12(9):701-4.

Kaminogawa S, Nanno M. Modulation of immune functions by foods. Evid Based Complement Alternat Med. 2004 Dec;1(3):241-250.

Kaaks R. Nutrition, insulin, IGF-1 metabolism and cancer risk: a summary of epidemiological evidence. Novartis Found Symp. 2004; 262:247-60.

Kaaks R, Bellati C, Venturelli E et al. Effects of dietary intervention on IGF-I and IGF-binding proteins, and related alterations in sex steroid metabolism: the Diet and Androgens (DIANA) Randomised Trial. Eur J Clin Nutr. 2003 Sep;57(9):1079-88.

Kall MA, Vang O, Clausen J. Effects of dietary broccoli on human in vivo drug metabolizing enzymes: evaluation of caffeine, oestrone and chlorzoxazone metabolism. Carcinogenesis. 1996;17(4):793-9.

Kasper JS, Liu Y, Pollak MN, Rifai N, Giovannucci E. Hormonal profile of diabetic men and the potential link to prostate cancer. Cancer Causes Control. 2008 Sep;19(7):703-10.

Kazimirova A, Barancokova M, Volkovova K et al. Does a vegetarian diet influence genomic stability? Eur J Nutr. 2004 Feb;43(1):32-8.

Kennedy DO, Agrawal M, Shen J et al. DNA repair capacity of lymphoblastoid cell lines from sisters discordant for breast cancer. J Natl Cancer Inst. 2005 Jan 19;97(2):127-32.

Kesteloot H, Lesaffre E, Joossens JV. Dairy fat, saturated animal fat, and cancer risk. *Prev Med.* 1991;20:226- 36.

Kirschner MA, Ertel N, Schneider G. Obesity, hormones, and cancer. Cancer Res. 1981 Sep;41(9 Pt 2):3711-7.

Koutros S, Cross AJ, Sandler DP et al. Meat and meat mutagens and risk of prostate cancer in the Agricultural Health Study. Cancer Epidemiol Biomarkers Prev. 2008 Jan;17:80-7.

Krajcovicova-Kudlackova M, Dusinska M. Oxidative DNA damage in relation to nutrition. Neoplasma 2004;51(1):30-3.

Krajcovicová-Kudláčková M, Valachovicová M, Pauková V, Dusinská M. Effects of diet and age on oxidative damage products in healthy subjects. Physiol Res. 2008;57(4):647-51.

Kumar N, Allen K, Riccardi D, Kazi A, Heine J. Isoflavones in breast cancer chemoprevention: where do we go from here? Front Biosci. 2004 Sep 1;9:2927-34.

Kurahashi N, Inoue M, Iwasaki M, Sasazuki S, Tsugane AS; Japan Public Health Center-Based Prospective Study Group. Dairy product, saturated fatty acid, and calcium intake and prostate cancer in a prospective cohort of Japanese men. Cancer Epidemiol Biomarkers Prev. 2008 Apr;17(4):930-7.

Lampe JW. Diet, genetic polymorphisms, detoxification, and health risks. Altern Ther Health Med. 2007 Mar-Apr;13(2):S108-11.

Lampe JW, Chen C, Li S, et al. Modulation of human glutathione S-transferases by botanically defined vegetable diets. Cancer Epidemiol Biomarkers Prev. 2000 Aug;9(8):787-93.

Larsson SC, Bergkvist L, Wolk A. Milk and lactose intakes and ovarian cancer risk in the Swedish Mammography Cohort. *Am J Clin Nutr.* 2004;80:1353-7.

La Vecchia C, Chatenoud L. Fibres, whole-grain foods and breast and other cancers. Eur J Cancer Prev. 1998 May;7 Suppl 2:S25-8.

Lee JH, O'Keefe JH, Bell D, Hensrud DD, Holick MF. Vitamin D deficiency an important, common, and easily treatable cardiovascular risk factor? J Am Coll Cardiol. 2008 Dec 9;52(24):1949-56.

Lee SA, Fowke JH, Lu W et al. Cruciferous vegetables, the GSTP1 Ile105Val genetic polymorphism, and breast cancer risk. Am J Clin Nutr. 2008 Mar;87(3):753-60.

Lee SY, Shin YW, Hahm KB. Phytoceuticals: mighty but ignored weapons against Helicobacter pylori infection. J Dig Dis. 2008 Aug;9(3):129-39.

LeRoith D, Novosyadlyy R, Gallagher EJ, Lann D, Vijayakumar A, Yakar S. Obesity and type 2 diabetes are associated with an increased risk of developing cancer and a worse prognosis; epidemiological and mechanistic evidence. Exp Clin Endocrinol Diabetes. 2008 Sep;116 Suppl 1:S4-6.

Li C, Wang LE, Wei Q. DNA repair phenotype and cancer susceptibility--a mini review. Int J Cancer. 2009 Mar 1;124(5):999-1007.

Li D, Wang M, Dhingra K, Hittelman WN. Aromatic DNA adducts in adjacent tissues of breast cancer patients: clues to breast cancer etiology. Cancer Res. 1996 Jan 15;56(2):287-93.

Loft S, Møller P, Cooke MS, Rozalski R, Olinski R. Antioxidant vitamins and cancer risk: is oxidative damage to DNA a relevant biomarker? Eur J Nutr. 2008 May;47 Suppl 2:19-28.

Loft S, Vistisen K, Ewertz M, Tjonneland A, Overvad K, Poulsen HE et al. Oxidative DNA damage estimated by 8-hydroxydeoxyguanosine excretion in humans: influence of smoking, gender and body mass index. Carcinogenesis. 1992 Dec;13(12):2241-7.

Lucia MS, Torkko KC. Inflammation as a target for prostate cancer chemoprevention: pathological and laboratory rationale. J Urol. 2004 Feb;171(2 Pt 2):S30-4.

Lukanova A, Zeleniuch-Jacquotte A, Lundin E et al. Prediagnostic levels of C-peptide, IGF-I, IGFBP -1, -2 and risk of endometrial cancer. Int J Cancer. 2004 Jan 10;108(2):262-8.

Ma J, Giovannucci E, Pollak M, Chan JM, Gaziano JM, Willett W, Stampfer MJ. Milk intake, circulating levels of insulin-like growth factor-I, and risk of colorectal cancer in men. J Natl Cancer Inst. 2001 Sep 5;93:1330-6.

Ma J, Giovannucci E, Pollak M, Leavitt A, Tao Y, Gaziano JM, Stampfer MJ. A prospective study of plasma C-peptide and colorectal cancer risk in men. J Natl Cancer Inst. 2004 Apr 7;96(7):546-53.

Ma J, Li H, Giovannucci E, Mucci L et al. Prediagnostic body-mass index, plasma C-peptide concentration, and prostate cancer-specific mortality in men with prostate cancer: a long-term survival analysis. Lancet Oncol. 2008 Nov;9(11):1039-47.

Majed B, Moreau T, Senouci K, Salmon RJ, Fourquet A, Asselain B. Is obesity an independent prognosis factor in woman breast cancer? Breast Cancer Res Treat. 2008 Sep;111(2):329-42.

Messina MJ. Emerging evidence on the role of soy in reducing prostate cancer risk. Nutr Rev. 2003; 61:117-31.

Mantzoros CS. The role of leptin in human obesity and disease: a review of current evidence. Ann Intern Med. 1999 Apr 20;130(8):671-80.

Magee PJ, Rowland IR. Phyto-oestrogens, their mechanism of action: current evidence for a role in breast and prostate cancer. Br J Nutr. 2004;91(4):513-31.

Malfertheiner P, Fry LC, Mönkemüller K. Can gastric cancer be prevented by Helicobacter pylori eradication? Best Pract Res Clin Gastroenterol. 2006;20(4):709-19.

Mandayam S, Shahinian VB. Are chronic dialysis patients at increased risk for cancer? J Nephrol. 2008 Mar-Apr;21(2):166-74.

Matsuo K, Hiraki A, Ito H et al. Soy consumption reduces the risk of non-small-cell lung cancers with epidermal growth factor receptor mutations among Japanese. Cancer Sci. 2008 Jun;99(6):1202-8.

McDougall J. Diet-induced precocious puberty. Accessed 6-26-2005 at: http://www.drmcdougall.com/newsletter/nov_dec97.html

McKeown NM, Meigs JB, Liu S, Saltzman E, Wilson PW, Jacques PF. Carbohydrate nutrition, insulin resistance, and the prevalence of the metabolic syndrome in the Framingham Offspring Cohort. Diabetes Care 2004 Feb;27(2):538-46.

McMichael AJ, Powles JW, Butler CD, Uauy R. Food, livestock production, energy, climate change, and health. Lancet. 2007 Oct 6;370(9594):1253-63.

McTiernan A. Behavioral risk factors in breast cancer: can risk be modified? *Oncologist.* 2003; 8(4):326-334.

Menendez JA, Lupu R. Mediterranean dietary traditions for the molecular treatment of human cancer: anti-oncogenic actions of the main olive oil's monounsaturated fatty acid oleic acid (18:1n-9). Curr Pharm Biotechnol. 2006 Dec;7(6):495-502.

Mettlin C. Milk drinking, other beverage habits, and lung cancer risk. *Int J Cancer.* 1989;43:608-12. Michaud DS, Augustsson K, Rimm EB, Stampfer MJ, Willet WC, Giovannucci E. A prospective study on intake of animal products and risk of prostate cancer. Cancer Causes Control. 2001 Aug;12(6):557-67.

Miller K. Estrogen and DNA damage: the silent source of breast cancer? J Natl Cancer Inst. 2003;95(2):100-2.

Moller P, Vogel U, Pedersen A, Dragsted LO, Sandstrom B, Loft S. No effect of 600 grams fruit and vegetables per day on oxidative DNA damage and repair in healthy nonsmokers. Cancer Epidemiol Biomarkers Prev. 2003 Oct;12(10):1016-22.

Monroe KR, Murphy SP, Henderson BE, Kolonel LN, Stanczyk FZ, Adlercreutz H, Pike MC. Dietary fiber intake and endogenous serum hormone levels in naturally postmenopausal Mexican American women: the Multiethnic Cohort Study. Nutr Cancer. 2007;58(2):127-35.

Morisset AS, Blouin K, Tchernof A. Impact of diet and adiposity on circulating levels of sex hormone-binding globulin and androgens. Nutr Rev. 2008 Sep;66(9):506-16.

Moskaug JØ, Carlsen H, Myhrstad MC, Blomhoff R. Polyphenols and glutathione synthesis regulation. Am J Clin Nutr. 2005 Jan;81(1 Suppl):277S-283S.

Nagata C, Nagao Y, Shibuya C, Kashiki Y, Shimizu H. Association of vegetable intake with urinary 6-sulfatoxymelatonin level. Cancer Epidemiol Biomarkers Prev. 2005 May;14(5):1333-5.

Naumov GN, Akslen LA, Folkman J. Role of angiogenesis in human tumor dormancy: animal models of the angiogenic switch. Cell Cycle. 2006 Aug;5(16):1779-87.

Nestle M. *Food Politics: How the Food Industry Influences Nutrition and Health.* Berkeley, CA: University of California Press, 2002.

Ngata C, Shimizu H, Takami R, Hayashi M, Takeda N, Yasuda K. Dietary soy and fats in relation to serum insulin-like growth factor-1 and insulin-like growth factor-binding protein-3 levels in premenopausal Japanese women. Nutr Cancer. 2003;45(2):185-9.

Nohmi T, Kim SR, Yamada M. Modulation of oxidative mutagenesis and carcinogenesis by polymorphic forms of human DNA repair enzymes. Mutat Res. 2005 Dec 11;591(1-2):60-73.

O'Rourke RW. Inflammation in obesity-related diseases. Surgery. 2009 Mar;145(3):255-9.

Pérez DD, Strobel P, Foncea R et al. Wine, diet, antioxidant defenses, and oxidative damage. Ann N Y Acad Sci. 2002 May;957:136-45.

Pierce JP, Natarajan L, Caan BJ et al. Influence of a diet very high in vegetables, fruit, and fiber and low in fat on prognosis following treatment for breast cancer: the Women's Healthy Eating and Living (WHEL) randomized trial. JAMA. 2007 Jul 18;298(3):289-98.

Philpott M, Ferguson LR. Immunonutrition and cancer. Mutat Res. 2004 Jul 13;551(1-2):29-42.

Pool-Zobel BL, Bub A, Liegibel UM, Treptow-van Lishaut S, Rechkemmer G. Mechanisms by which vegetable consumption reduces genetic damage in humans. Cancer Epidemiol Biomarkers Prev. 1998 Oct;7(10):891-9.

Pierce JP, Stefanick ML, Flatt SW et al. Greater survival after breast cancer in physically active women with high vegetable-fruit intake regardless of obesity. J Clin Oncol. 2007 Jun 10;25(17):2345-51.

Platz EA. Energy imbalance and prostate cancer. J Nutr. 2002 Nov; 132(11 Suppl):3471S-3481S.

Prins GS. Endocrine disruptors and prostate cancer risk. Endocr Relat Cancer. 2008 Sep;15(3):649-56.

Probst-Hensch NM, Wang H, Goh VH, Seow A, Lee HP, Yu MC. Determinants of circulating insulin-like growth factor I and insulin-like growth factor binding protein 3 concentrations in a cohort of Singapore men and women. Cancer Epidemiol Biomarkers Prev. 2003 Aug;12:739-46.

Rarick KR, Pikosky MA, Grediagin A et alEnergy flux, more so than energy balance, protein intake, or fitness level, influences insulin-like growth factor-I system responses during 7 days of increased physical activity. J Appl Physiol. 2007 Nov;103(5):1613-21.

Ravaglia G, Forti P, Maioli F et al. Effect of micronutrient status on natural killer cell immune function in healthy free-living subjects aged >/=90 y. Am J Clin Nutr. 2000 Feb;71(2):590-8.

Reinehr T, de Sousa G, Roth CL, Andler W. Androgens before and after weight loss in obese children. J Clin Endocrinol Metab. 2005 Oct;90(10):5588-95.

Renehan AG, Tyson M, Egger M, Heller RF, Zwahlen M. Body-mass index and incidence of cancer: a systematic review and meta-analysis of prospective observational studies. Lancet. 2008;371(9612):569-78. Reiter RJ, Manchester LC, Tan DX. Melatonin in walnuts: Influence on levels of melatonin and total antioxidant capacity of blood. Nutrition. 2005 Sep;21(9):920-4.

Rich-Edwards JW, Ganmaa D et al. Milk consumption and the prepubertal somatotropic axis. Nutr J. 2007 Sep 27;6:28.

Renehan AG, Zwahlen M, Minder C, O'Dwyer ST, Shalet SM, Egger M. Insulin-like growth factor (IGF)-I, IGF binding protein-3, and cancer risk: systematic review and meta-regression analysis. Lancet. 2004 Apr 24;363(9418):1346-53.

Rock CL, Flatt SW, Thomson CA el. Effects of a high-fiber, low-fat diet intervention on serum concentrations of reproductive steroid hormones in women with a history of breast cancer. J Clin Oncol. 2004 Jun 15;22(12):2379-87.

Roddam AW, Allen NE, Appleby P et al. Insulin-like growth factors, their binding proteins, and prostate cancer risk: analysis of individual patient data from 12 prospective studies. Ann Intern Med. 2008;149(7):461-71.

Rogers CJ, Colbert LH, Greiner JW, Perkins SN, Hursting SD. Physical activity and cancer prevention : pathways and targets for intervention. Sports Med. 2008;38(4):271-96.

Rose DP, Gilhooly EM, Nixon DW. Adverse effects of obesity on breast cancer prognosis, and the biological actions of leptin (review). Int J Oncol. 2002 Dec;21(6):1285-92.

Rose DP, Komninou D, Stephenson GD. Obesity, adipocytokines, and insulin resistance in breast cancer. Obes Rev. 2004 Aug;5(3):153-65.

Rose DP, Cohen LA, Berke B, Boyar AP. Effect of a low-fat diet on hormone levels in women with cystic breast disease. II. Serum radioimmunoassayable prolactin and growth hormone and bioactive lactogenic hormones. J Natl Cancer Inst. 1987 Apr;78(4):627-31.

Ross JK, Pusateri DJ, Shultz TD. Dietary and hormonal evaluation of men at different risks for prostate cancer: fiber intake, excretion, and composition, with in vitro evidence for an association between steroid hormones and specific fiber components. Am J Clin Nutr. 1990 Mar,51(3):365-70

Samet JM, Geyh AS, Utell MJ. The legacy of World Trade Center dust N Engl J Med. 2007 May 31;356(22):2233-6.

Sánchez-Chapado M, Olmedilla G, Cabeza M, Donat E, Ruiz A. Prevalence of prostate cancer and prostatic intraepithelial neoplasia in Caucasian Mediterranean males: an autopsy study. Prostate. 2003;54(3):238-47.

Santner SJ, Albertson B, Zhang GY et al. Comparative rates of androgen production and metabolism in Caucasian and Chinese subjects. J Clin Endocrinol Metab. 1998 Jun;83(6):2104-9.

Santos MS, Gaziano JM, Leka LS, Beharka AA, Hennekens CH, Meydani SN. Beta-carotene-induced enhancement of natural killer cell activity in elderly men: an investigation of the role of cytokines. Am J Clin Nutr. 1998 Jul;68(1):164-70.

Saxe GA, Rock CL, Wicha MS, Schottenfeld D. Diet and risk for breast cancer recurrence and survival. Breast Cancer Res Treat. 1999 Feb;53(3):241-53.

Schecter A, Wallace D, Pavuk M, Piskac A, Päpke O. Dioxins in commercial United States baby food. J Toxicol Environ Health A. 2002 Dec 13;65(23):1937-43.

Schernhammer ES, Berrino F, Krogh V et al. Urinary 6-sulfatoxymelatonin levels and risk of breast cancer in postmenopausal women. J Natl Cancer Inst. 2008 Jun 18;100(12):898-905.

Schernhammer ES, Hu FB, Giovannucci E et al. Sugar-sweetened soft drink consumption and risk of pancreatic cancer in two prospective cohorts. Cancer Epidemiol Biomarkers Prev. 2005; 14(9):2098-105. Schernhammer ES, Kroenke CH, Dowsett M, Folkerd E, Hankinson SE. Urinary 6-sulfatoxymelatonin levels and their correlations with lifestyle factors and steroid hormone levels. J Pineal Res. 2006 Mar;40(2):116-24.

Schwalfenberg G. Not enough vitamin D: health consequences for Canadians. Can Fam Physician. 2007

May;53(5):841-54.

Schouten LJ, Rivera C, Hunter DJ et al. Height, body mass index, and ovarian cancer: a pooled analysis of 12 cohort studies. Cancer Epidemiol Biomarkers Prev. 2008 Apr;17(4):902-12.

Sen CK, Packer L. Antioxidant and redox regulation of gene transcription. *FASEB J.* 1996; 10: 709–720.

Setlow RB. Human cancer: etiologic agents/dose responses/DNA repair/cellular and animal models. Mutat Res. 2001 Jun 2;477(1-2):1-6.

Sharman MJ, Volek JS. Weight loss leads to reductions in inflammatory biomarkers after a very-low-carbohydrate diet and a low-fat diet in overweight men. Clin Sci (Lond). 2004 Oct;107(4):365-9.

Silha JV, Krsek M, Sucharda P, Murphy LJ. Angiogenic factors are elevated in overweight and obese individuals. Int J Obes (Lond). 2005 Nov;29(11):1308-14.

Sinha R, Kulldorff M, Curtin J, Brown CC, Alavanja MC, Swanson CA. Fried, well-done red meat and risk of lung cancer in women (United States). Cancer Causes Control. 1998 Dec;9(6):621-30.

Sivakumar B, Harry LE, Paleolog EM. Modulating angiogenesis: more vs. less. JAMA. 2004 Aug 25; 292(8):972-7.

Sorensen M, Autrup H, Moller P et al. Linking exposure to environmental pollutants with biological effects. Mutat Res. 2003 Nov;544(2-3):255-71.

Sofi F, Cesari F, Abbate R, Gensini GF, Casini A. Adherence to Mediterranean diet and health status: meta-analysis. BMJ. 2008 Sep 11;337:a1344. doi: 10.1136/bmj.a1344.

Soto AM, Vandenberg LN, Maffini MV, Sonnenschein C. Does breast cancer start in the womb? Basic Clin Pharmacol Toxicol. 2008 Feb;102(2):125-33.

Sottero B, Gamba P, Gargiulo S, Leonarduzzi G, Poli G. Cholesterol oxidation products and disease: an emerging topic of interest in medicinal chemistry. Curr Med Chem. 2009;16(6):685-705.

Spector D, Anthony M, Alexander D, Arab L. Soy consumption and colorectal cancer. Nutr Cancer.2003;47(1):1

Spira AI, Carducci MA. Differentiation therapy. Curr Opin Pharmacol. 2003 Aug;3(4):338-43.

Spitz MR, Duphorne CM, Detry MA et al. Dietary intake of isothiocyanates: evidence of a joint effect with glutathione S-transferase polymorphisms in lung cancer risk. Cancer Epid Biomarkers Prev. 2000; 9:1017-20.

Starek A. Estrogens and organochlorine xenoestrogens and breast cancer risk. Int J Occup Med Environ Health. 2003;16(2):113-24.

Stroescu V, Dragan J, Simionescu L, Stroescu OV. Hormonal and metabolic response in elite female gymnasts undergoing strenuous training and supplementation with SUPRO Brand Isolated Soy Protein. J Sports Med Phys Fitness. 2001 Mar;41(1):89-94.

Sugimura T, Wakabayashi K, Nakagama H, Nagao M. Heterocyclic amines: Mutagens/carcinogens produced during cooking of meat and fish. Cancer Sci. 2004 Apr;95(4):290-9.

Terry KL, Willett WC, Rich-Edwards JW, Michels KB. Menstrual cycle characteristics and incidence of premenopausal breast cancer. Cancer Epidemiol Biomarkers Prev. 2005 Jun;14(6):1509-13.

Thessaloniki ESHRE/ASRM-Sponsored PCOS Consensus Workshop Group. Consensus on infertility treatment related to polycystic ovary syndrome. Consensus on infertility treatment related to polycystic ovary syndrome. Hum Reprod. 2008 Mar;23(3):462-77. doi: 10.1093/humrep/dem426.

Thiébaut AC, Schatzkin A, Ballard-Barbash R, Kipnis V. Dietary fat and breast cancer: contributions from a survival trial. J Natl Cancer Inst. 2006 Dec 20;98(24):1753-5.

Thomson CA, Giuliano AR, Shaw JW et al. Diet and biomarkers of oxidative damage in women previously treated for breast cancer. Nutr Cancer. 2005;51(2):146-54.

Thompson HJ, Zhu Z, Jiang W. Weight control and breast cancer prevention: are the effects of reduced energy intake equivalent to those of increased energy expenditure? J Nutr. 2004;134(12 Suppl):3407S-3411S.

Tomlinson JW, Finney J, Hughes BA, Hughes SV, Stewart PM. Reduced glucocorticoid production rate, decreased 5alpha-reductase activity, and adipose tissue insulin sensitization after weight loss. Diabetes. 2008;57(6):1536-43.

Tosetti F, Ferrari N, De Flora S, Albini A. 'Angioprevention': angiogenesis is a common and key target for cancer chemopreventive agents. FASEB J. 2002 Jan; 16(1):2-14.

Traka M, Gasper AV, Melchini A et al. Broccoli consumption interacts with GSTM1 to perturb oncogenic signaling pathways in the prostate. PLoS ONE. 2008 Jul 2;3(7):e2568.

Tudek B, Swoboda M, Kowalczyk P, Oliński R. Modulation of oxidative DNA damage repair by the diet, inflammation and neoplastic transformation. J Physiol Pharmacol. 2006 Nov;57 Suppl 7:33-49.

Tymchuk CN, Tessler SB, Barnard RJ. Changes in sex hormone-binding globulin, insulin, and serum lipids in postmenopausal women on a low-fat, high-fiber diet combined with exercise. Nutr Cancer. 2000;38(2):158-62.

Ursin G, Bjelke E, Heuch I, Vollset SE. Milk consumption and cancer incidence: a Norwegian prospective study. *Br J Cancer.* 1990;61:456-9.

Utz PJ, Gensler TJ, Anderson P. Death, autoantigen modifications, and tolerance. Arthritis Res. 2000;2:101-14.

van Dam RM, Li T, Spiegelman D, Franco OH, Hu FB. Combined impact of lifestyle factors on mortality: prospective cohort study in US women. BMJ. 2008 Sep 16;337:a1440.

van Houten ME, Gooren LJ. Differences in reproductive endocrinology between Asian men and Caucasian men--a literature review. Asian J Androl. 2000 Mar;2(1):13-20.

Van Maele-Fabry G, Libotte V, Willems J, Lison D. Review and meta-analysis of risk estimates for prostate cancer in pesticide manufacturing workers. Cancer Causes Control. 2006 May;17(4):353-73.

Velie EM, Nechuta S, Osuch JR. Lifetime reproductive and anthropometric risk factors for breast cancer in postmenopausal women. Breast Dis. 2005-2006;24:17-35.

Villanueva CM, Fernández F, Malats N, Grimalt JO, Kogevinas M. Meta-analysis of studies on individual consumption of chlorinated drinking water and bladder cancer. J Epidemiol Community Health. 2003 Mar;57(3):166-73.

Vina J, Borras C, Gambini J, Sastre J, Pallardo FV. Why females live longer than males: control of longevity by sex hormones. Sci Aging Knowledge Environ. 2005 8;2005(23):pe17.

Vina J, Sastre J, Pallardo F, Borras C. Mitochondrial theory of aging: importance to explain why females live longer than males. Antioxid Redox Signal. 2003;5(5):549-56.

Vineis P, Forastiere F, Hoek G, Lipsett M. Outdoor air pollution and lung cancer: recent epidemiologic evidence. Int J Cancer. 2004 Sep 20;111(5):647-52.

Viswanathan AN, Schernhammer ES. Circulating melatonin and the risk of breast and endometrial cancer in women. Cancer Lett. 2009 Aug 18;281(1):1-7.

Vona-Davis L, Rose DP. Adipokines as endocrine, paracrine, and autocrine factors in breast cancer risk and progression. Endocr Relat Cancer. 2007 Jun;14(2):189-206.

Wang C, Catlin DH, Starcevic B et al. Low-fat high-fiber diet decreased serum and urine androgens in men. J Clin Endocrinol Metab. 2005 Jun;90(6):3550-9.

Wang J, John EM, Ingles SA. 5-lipoxygenase and 5-lipoxygenase-activating protein gene polymorphisms, dietary linoleic acid, and risk for breast cancer. Cancer Epidemiol Biomarkers Prev. 2008;17(10):2748-54.

Wang XD, Liu C, Chung J, Stickel F, Seitz HK, Russell RM. Chronic alcohol intake reduces retinoic acid concentration and enhances AP-1 (c-Jun and c-Fos) expression in rat liver. Hepatology. 1998 Sep;28(3):744-50.

Wang Z. DNA damage-induced mutagenesis : a novel target for cancer prevention. Mol Interv. 2001;1(5):269-81.

Wayne SJ, Neuhouser ML, Ulrich CM et al. Dietary fiber is associated with serum sex hormones and insulin-related peptides in postmenopausal breast cancer survivors. Breast Cancer Res Treat. 2008 Nov;112(1):149-58.

WCRF/AICR *Food, Nutrition, Physical Activity and the Prevention of Cancer: A Global Perspective.* Washington, D.C.: AICR, 2007.

Weihrauch MR, Diehl V. Artificial sweeteners—do they bear a carcinogenic risk? Ann Oncol. 2004 Oct;15(10):1460-5.

Whittemore AS, Kolonel LN, Wu AH et al. Prostate cancer in relation to diet, physical activity, and body size in blacks, whites, and Asians in the United States and Canada. J Natl Cancer Inst. 1995 May 3;87(9):652-61.

Wigle DT, Turner MC, Gomes J, Parent ME. Role of hormonal and other factors in human prostate cancer. J Toxicol Environ Health B Crit Rev. 2008 Mar;11(3-4):242-59.

Wiley AS. Does milk make children grow? Relationships between milk consumption and height in NHANES 1999-2002 Am J Hum Biol. 2005 Jul-Aug;17(4):425-41.

Wilt TJ, MacDonald R, Hagerty K et al. Five-alpha-reductase Inhibitors for prostate cancer prevention. Cochrane Database Syst Rev. 2008 Apr 16;(2):CD007091.

Wogan GN, Hecht SS, Felton JS, Conney AH, Loeb LA. Environmental and chemical carcinogenesis. Semin Cancer Biol. 2004 Dec;14(6):473-86.

Xiao X, Xiong A, Chen X, Mao X, Zhou X. Epidermal growth factor concentrations in human milk, cow's milk and cow's milk-based infant formulas. Chin Med J (Engl). 2002 Mar;115(3):451-4.

Yagi H, Suzuki S, Noji T, Nagashima K, Kuroume T. Epidermal growth factor in cow's milk and milk formulas. Acta Paediatr Scand. 1986 Mar;75(2):233-5.

Yang CS, Landau JM. Effects of tea consumption on nutrition and health. J Nutr. 2000;130(10):2409-12.

Yin L, Grandi N, Raum E, Haug U, Arndt V, Brenner H. Meta-analysis: longitudinal studies of serum vitamin D and colorectal cancer risk. Aliment Pharmacol Ther. 2009 Jul 1;30(2):113-25.

Zhao B, Seow A, Lee EJ et al.. Dietary isothiocyanates, glutathione S-transferase -M1, -T1 polymorphisms and lung cancer risk among Chinese women in Singapore. Cancer Epidemiol Biomarkers Prev. 2001; 10(10):1063-7.

Zheng W, Lee SA. Well-done meat intake, heterocyclic amine exposure, and cancer risk. Nutr Cancer. 2009;61(4):437-46.

Zi X, Singh RP, Agarwal R. Impairment of erbB1 receptor and fluid-phase endocytosis and associated mitogenic signaling by inositol hexaphosphate in human prostate carcinoma DU145 cells. Carcinogenesis. 2000;21:2225-35.

Ziccardi P, Nappo F, Giugliano G et al. Reduction of inflammatory cytokine concentrations and improvement of endothelial functions in obese women after weight loss over one year. Circulation. 2002 Feb 19;105(7):804-9.

Zisman TL, Rubin DT. Colorectal cancer and dysplasia in inflammatory bowel disease. World J Gastroenterol. 2008 May 7;14(17):2662-9.

Zive MM, Nicklas TA, Busch EC, Myers L, Berenson GS. Marginal vitamin and mineral intakes of young adults: the Bogalusa Heart Study. J Adolescent Health 1996; 19:39-47.

Zwiener C, Richardson SD, DeMarini DM, Grummt T, Glauner T, Frimmel FH. Drowning in disinfection by-products? Assessing swimming pool water. Environ Sci Technol. 2007 Jan 15;41(2):363-72.

Thornburg KL, Shannon J, Thuillier P, Turker MS. In utero life and epigenetic predisposition for disease. Adv Genet. 2010;71:57-78.

Xu X, Dailey AB, Peoples-Sheps M, Talbott EO, Li N, Roth J. Birth weight as a risk factor for breast cancer: a meta-analysis of 18 epidemiological studies. J Womens Health (Larchmt). 2009 Aug;18(8):1169-78.

References: Chapter Two: Soy Foods: Your # 1 friend in the cancer battle

Adams KF, Chen C, Newton KM, Potter JD, Lampe JW. Soy isoflavones do not modulate prostate-specific antigen concentrations in older men in a randomized controlled trial.Cancer Epidemiol Biomarkers Prev. 2004;13:644-8.

Constantinou A, Huberman E. Genistein as an inducer of tumor cell differentiation: possible mechanisms of action. Proc Soc Exp Biol Med. 1995 Jan;208(1):109-15.

Constantinou AI, Krygier AE, Mehta RR. Genistein induces maturation of cultured human breast cancer cells and prevents tumor growth in nude mice. Am J Clin Nutr. 1998 Dec;68(6 Suppl):1426S-1430S.

Cook KM, Figg WD. Angiogenesis inhibitors: current strategies and future prospects. CA Cancer J Clin. 2010 Jul-Aug;60(4):222-43.

Cuzick J, Otto F, Baron JA, Brown PH, Burn J, Greenwald P, Jankowski J, La Vecchia C, Meyskens F, Senn HJ, Thun M. Aspirin and non-steroidal anti-inflammatory drugs for cancer prevention: an international consensus statement. Lancet Oncol. 2009 May;10(5):501-7.

Dewell A, Weidner G, Sumner MD et al. Relationship of dietary protein and soy isoflavones to serum IGF-1 and IGF binding proteins in the Prostate Cancer Lifestyle Trial. Nutr Cancer. 2007;58(1):35-42.

Dillingham BL, McVeigh BL, Lampe JW, Duncan AM. Soy protein isolates of varying isoflavone content exert minor effects on serum reproductive hormones in healthy young men. J Nutr. 2005 Mar;135(3):584-91.

Dip R, Lenz S, Antignac JP, Le Bizec B, Gmuender H, Naegeli H. Global gene expression profiles induced by phytoestrogens in human breast cancer cells. Endocr Relat Cancer. 2008 Mar;15(1):161-73.

Dou QP, Li B. Proteasome inhibitors as potential novel anticancer agents. Drug Resist Updat. 1999 Aug;2(4):215-223.

Giannini S, Serio M, Galli A. Pleiotropic effects of thiazolidinediones: taking a look beyond antidiabetic activity. J Endocrinol Invest. 2004 Nov;27(10):982-91.

Grainger EM, Schwartz SJ, Wang S, Unlu NZ, Boileau TW, Ferketich AK, Monk JP, Gong MC, Bahnson RR, DeGroff VL, Clinton SK. A combination of tomato and soy products for men with recurring prostate cancer and rising prostate specific antigen. Nutr Cancer. 2008;60(2):145-54.

Green S, Furr B. Prospects for the treatment of endocrine-responsive tumours. Endocr Relat Cancer. 1999 Sep;6(3):349-71.

Hamilton-Reeves JM, Rebello SA, Thomas W, Slaton JW, Kurzer MS. Isoflavone-rich soy protein isolate suppresses androgen receptor expression without altering estrogen receptor-beta expression or serum hormonal profiles in men at high risk of prostate cancer. J Nutr. 2007 Jul;137(7):1769-75.

Hannun YA, Linardic CM. Sphingolipid breakdown products: anti-proliferative and tumor-suppressor lipids. Biochim Biophys Acta. 1993 Dec 21;1154(3-4):223-36.

Hardman WE. Omega-3 fatty acids to augment cancer therapy. J Nutr. 2002 Nov;132(11 Suppl):3508S-3512S.

Interview with Dr. Ivana Vucenik, 1-12-06.

Hargreaves DF, Potten CS, Harding C, Shaw LE, Morton MS, Roberts SA, Howell A, Bundred NJ. Two-week dietary soy supplementation has an estrogenic effect on normal premenopausal breast. J Clin Endocrinol Metab. 1999 Nov;84(11):4017-24.

Hooper L, Madhavan G, Tice JA, Leinster SJ, Cassidy A. Effects of isoflavones on breast density in pre- and post-menopausal women: a systematic review and meta-analysis of randomized controlled trials. Hum Reprod Update. 2010 Nov-Dec;16(6):745-60.

Hussain M, Banerjee M, Sarkar FH et al. Soy isoflavones in the treatment of prostate cancer. Nutr Cancer. 2003;47(2):111-7.

Interview with Dr. Coral Lamartiniere 1-4-06.

Joniau S, Goeman L, Roskams T, Lerut E, Oyen R, Van Poppel H. Effect of nutritional supplement challenge in patients with isolated high-grade prostatic intraepithelial neoplasia. Urology. 2007 Jun;69(6):1102-6.

Jones JL, Daley BJ, Enderson BL, Zhou JR, Karlstad MD. Genistein inhibits tamoxifen effects on cell proliferation and cell cycle arrest in T47D breast cancer cells. Am Surg. 2002 Jun;68(6):575-7.

Kwan W, Duncan G, Van Patten C, Liu M, Lim J. A phase II trial of a soy beverage for subjects without clinical disease with rising prostate-specific antigen after radical radiation for prostate cancer. Nutr Cancer. 2010;62:198-207.

Kazi A, Daniel KG, Smith DM, Kumar NB, Dou QP. Inhibition of the proteasome activity, a novel mechanism associated with the tumor cell apoptosis-inducing ability of genistein. Biochem Pharmacol. 2003;66:965-76.

Kelly RJ, Lopez-Chavez A, Citrin D, Janik JE, Morris JC. Impacting tumor cell-fate by targeting the inhibitor of apoptosis protein survivin. Mol Cancer. 2011 Apr 6;10:35.

Lamartiniere CA. Timing of exposure and mammary cancer risk. J Mammary Gland Biol Neoplasia. 2002 Jan;7(1):67-76.

Marks LS, Kojima M, Demarzo A, Heber D, Bostwick DG, Qian J, Dorey FJ, Veltri RW, Mohler JL, Partin AW. Prostate cancer in native Japanese and Japanese-American men: effects of dietary differences on prostatic tissue.Urology. 2004 Oct;64(4):765-71.

Maskarinec G, Morimoto Y, Conroy SM, Pagano IS, Franke AA. The volume of nipple aspirate fluid is not affected by 6 months of treatment with soy foods in premenopausal women. J Nutr. 2011 Apr 1;141(4):626-30.

Ogawara H, Akiyama T, Ishida J, Watanabe S, Suzuki K. A specific inhibitor for tyrosine protein kinase from Pseudomonas. J Antibiot (Tokyo). 1986 Apr;39(4):606-8.

Petrakis NL, Barnes S, King EB, Lowenstein J, Wiencke J, Lee MM, Miike R, Kirk M, Coward L. Stimulatory influence of soy protein isolate on breast secretion in pre- and postmenopausal women. Cancer Epidemiol Biomarkers Prev. 1996 Oct;5(10):785-94.

Qin LQ, Xu JY, Wang PY, Hoshi K. Soyfood intake in the prevention of breast cancer risk in women: a meta-analysis of observational epidemiological studies. J Nutr Sci Vitaminol (Tokyo). 2006 Dec;52(6):428-36.

Ricketts ML, Moore DD, Banz WJ, Mezei O, Shay NF. Molecular mechanisms of action of the soy isoflavones includes activation of promiscuous nuclear receptors. A review. J Nutr Biochem. 2005 Jun;16(6):321-30.

Sartippour MR, Rao JY, Apple S, Wu D, Henning S, Wang H, Elashoff R, Rubio R, Heber D, Brooks MN. A pilot clinical study of short-term isoflavone supplements in breast cancer patients. Nutr Cancer. 2004;49:59-65.

Saxe GA, Hebert JR, Carmody JF, Kabat-Zinn J, Rosenzweig PH, Jarzobski D, Reed GW, Blute RD. Can diet in conjunction with stress reduction affect the rate of increase in prostate specific antigen after biochemical recurrence of prostate cancer? J Urol. 2001 Dec;166(6):2202-7.

Shu XO, Zheng Y, Cai H, Gu K, Chen Z, Zheng W, Lu W. Soy food intake and breast cancer survival. JAMA. 2009 Dec 9;302(22):2437-43.

Spentzos D, Mantzoros C, Regan MM, Morrissey ME, Duggan S, Flickner-Garvey S, McCormick H, DeWolf W, Balk S, Bubley GJ. Minimal effect of a low-fat/high soy diet for asymptomatic, hormonally naive prostate cancer patients. Clin Cancer Res. 2003 Aug 15;9(9):3282-7.

Spira AI, Carducci MA. Differentiation therapy. Curr Opin Pharmacol. 2003 Aug;3(4):338-43.

Teas J, Hurley TG, Hebert JR, Franke AA, Sepkovic DW, Kurzer MS. Dietary seaweed modifies estrogen and phytoestrogen metabolism in healthy postmenopausal women. J Nutr. 2009 May;139(5):939-44.

Tanaka M, Fujimoto K, Chihara Y, Torimoto K, Yoneda T, Tanaka N, Hirayama A, Miyanaga N, Akaza H, Hirao Y. Isoflavone supplements stimulated the production of serum equol and decreased the serum dihydrotestosterone levels in healthy male volunteers. Prostate Cancer Prostatic Dis. 2009;12(3):247-52.

Trock BJ, Hilakivi-Clarke L, Clarke R. Meta-analysis of soy intake and breast cancer risk. J Natl Cancer Inst. 2006 Apr 5;98(7):459-71.

Wang S, DeGroff VL, Clinton SK. Tomato and soy polyphenols reduce insulin-like growth factor-I-stimulated rat prostate cancer cell proliferation and apoptotic resistance in vitro via inhibition of intracellular signaling pathways involving tyrosine kinase.J Nutr. 2003 Jul;133(7):2367-76.

Wang J, Eltoum IE, Lamartiniere CA. Genistein alters growth factor signaling in transgenic prostate model (TRAMP). Mol Cell Endocrinol. 2004 Apr 30;219(1-2):171-80.

Wu AH, Yu MC, Tseng CC, Pike MC. Epidemiology of soy exposures and breast cancer risk. Br J Cancer. 2008 Jan 15;98(1):9-14.
Yan L, Spitznagel EL. Soy consumption and prostate cancer risk in men: a revisit of a meta-analysis. Am J Clin Nutr. 2009 Apr;89(4):1155-63.
Younes M, Honma N. Estrogen receptor β. Arch Pathol Lab Med. 2011 Jan;135(1):63-6.
Zhou JR, Gugger ET, Tanaka T, Guo Y, Blackburn GL, Clinton SK. Soybean phytochemicals inhibit the growth of transplantable human prostate carcinoma and tumor angiogenesis in mice. J Nutr 1999; 129:1628-35.

References: Chapter Three: Green tea: the all-hulk, no bulk cancer fighter

Adhami VM, Ahmad N, Mukhtar H. Molecular targets for green tea in prostate cancer prevention. J Nutr. 2003; Jul;133(7 Suppl):2417S-2424S.
Bettuzzi S, Brausi M, Rizzi F, Castagnetti G, Peracchia G, Corti A. Chemoprevention of human prostate cancer by oral administration of green tea catechins in volunteers with high-grade prostate intraepithelial neoplasia: a preliminary report from a one-year proof-of-principle study. Cancer Res. 2006 Jan 15;66(2):1234-40.
Blagosklonny MV. Cell death beyond apoptosis. Leukemia (2000) 14, 1502–1508.
Brusselmans K, Vrolix R, Verhoeven G, Swinnen JV. Induction of cancer cell apoptosis by flavonoids is associated with their ability to inhibit fatty acid synthase activity. J Biol Chem. 2005 Feb 18;280(7):5636-45.
Dorai T, Aggarwal BB. Role of chemopreventive agents in cancer therapy. Cancer Lett. 2004;215:129-40.
Dou QP. Molecular mechanisms of green tea polyphenols. Nutr Cancer. 2009;61(6):827-35.
Ezzedine K, Latreille J, Kesse-Guyot E, Galan P, Hercberg S, Guinot C, Malvy D. Incidence of skin cancers during 5-year follow-up after stopping antioxidant vitamins and mineral supplementation. Eur J Cancer. 2010 Dec;46(18):3316-22.
Garbisa S, Sartor L, Biggin S, Salvato B, Benelli R, Albini A. Tumor gelatinases and invasion inhibited by the green tea flavanol epigallocatechin-3-gallate. Cancer. 2001 Feb 15; 91(4):822-32.
Hakim IA, Chow HH, Harris RB. Green tea consumption is associated with decreased DNA damage among GSTM1-positive smokers regardless of their hOGG1 genotype. J Nutr. 2008 Aug;138(8):1567S-1571S.
Henning SM, Aronson W, Niu Y et al. Tea polyphenols and theaflavins are present in prostate tissue of humans and mice after green and black tea consumption. J Nutr. 2006 Jul;136(7):1839-43.
Kari C, Chan TO, Rocha de Quadros M, Rodeck U. Targeting the Epidermal Growth Factor Receptor in Cancer: Apoptosis Takes Center Stage. Cancer Research 2003; 63: 1-5.
Katiyar SK. Green tea prevents non-melanoma skin cancer by enhancing DNA repair. Arch Biochem Biophys. 2011 Apr 15;508(2):152-8.
Katiyar SK, Vaid M, van Steeg H, Meeran SM. Green tea polyphenols prevent UV-induced immunosuppression by rapid repair of DNA damage and enhancement of nucleotide excision repair genes. Cancer Prev Res (Phila). 2010 Feb;3(2):179-89.
Kuo YC, Yu CL, Liu CY, Wang SF, Pan PC, Wu MT, Ho CK, Lo YS, Li Y, Christiani DC; Kaohsiung Leukemia Research Group. A population-based, case-control study of green tea consumption and leukemia risk in southwestern Taiwan. Cancer Causes Control. 2009 Feb;20(1):57-65.
Kuhajda FP. Fatty acid synthase and cancer: new application of an old pathway. Cancer Res. 2006 Jun 15;66(12):5977-80.
Kurahashi N, Sasazuki S, Iwasaki M, Inoue M, Tsugane S; JPHC Study Group. Green tea consumption and prostate cancer risk in Japanese men: a prospective study. Am J Epidemiol. 2008 Jan 1;167(1):71-7.
Lambert JD, Yang CS. Mechanisms of cancer prevention by tea constituents. J Nutr. 2003 Oct;133(10):3262S-3267S.
Liotta LA, Thorgeirsson UP, Garbisa S. Role of collagenases in tumor cell invasion. Cancer Metastasis Rev. 1982;1(4):277-88.
McLarty J, Bigelow RL, Smith M, Elmajian D, Ankem M, Cardelli JA. Tea polyphenols decrease serum levels of prostate-specific antigen, hepatocyte growth factor, and vascular endothelial growth factor in prostate cancer patients and inhibit production of hepatocyte growth factor and vascular endothelial growth factor in vitro. Cancer Prev Res (Phila). 2009 Jul;2(7):673-82.
Menendez JA, Ropero S, Mehmi I, Atlas E, Colomer R, Lupu R. Overexpression and hyperactivity of breast cancer-associated fatty acid synthase (oncogenic antigen-519) is insensitive to normal arachidonic fatty acid-induced suppression in lipogenic tissues but it is selectively inhibited by tumoricidal alpha-linolenic and gamma-linolenic

fatty acids: a novel mechanism by which dietary fat can alter mammary tumorigenesis. Int J Oncol. 2004 Jun;24(6):1369-83.

Nichols JA, Katiyar SK. Skin photoprotection by natural polyphenols: anti-inflammatory, antioxidant and DNA repair mechanisms. Arch Dermatol Res. 2010 Mar;302(2):71-83.

Notarnicola M, Pisanti S, Tutino V, Bocale D, Rotelli MT, Gentile A, Memeo V et al. Effects of olive oil polyphenols on fatty acid synthase gene expression and activity in human colorectal cancer cells. Genes Nutr. 2011 Feb;6(1):63-9.

Notarnicola M, Tutino V, Calvani M, Lorusso D, Guerra V, Caruso MG. Serum Levels of Fatty Acid Synthase in Colorectal Cancer Patients Are Associated with Tumor Stage. J Gastrointest Cancer. 2011 Jul 5.

Puig T, Relat J, Marrero PF, Haro D, Brunet J, Colomer R. Green tea catechin inhibits fatty acid synthase without stimulating carnitine palmitoyltransferase-1 or inducing weight loss in experimental animals. Anticancer Res. 2008 Nov-Dec;28(6A):3671-6.

Santosh K. Katiyar,[1,2] Mudit Vaid,[1] Harry van Steeg,[3] and Syed M. Meeran. Drinking Green Tea Prevents UV-Induced Immunosuppression by Rapid Repair of UV-Induced DNA Damage and Enhancement of Nucleotide Excision Repair Genes. Cancer Prev Res (Phila). 2010 February; 3(2): 179–189.

Shimizu M, Weinstein IB. Modulation of signal transduction by tea catechins and related phytochemicals. Mutat Res. 2005 Dec 11;591(1-2):147-60.

Stahl W, Sies H. Carotenoids and flavonoids contribute to nutritional protection against skin damage from sunlight. Mol Biotechnol. 2007 Sep;37(1):26-30.

Tang FY, Nguyen N, Meydani M. Green tea catechins inhibit VEGF-induced angiogenesis in vitro through suppression of VE-cadherin phosphorylation and inactivation of Akt molecule. Int J Cancer. 2003 Oct 10; 106(6):871-8.

Vecchini A, Ceccarelli V, Susta F, Caligiana P, Orvietani P, Binaglia L, Nocentini G et al. Dietary alpha-linolenic acid reduces COX-2 expression and induces apoptosis of hepatoma cells. J Lipid Res. 2004 Feb;45(2):308-16.

References: Chapter Four: Attack of the Killer Tomatoes – and Beyond

Ahmad SM, Haskell MJ, Raqib R, Stephensen CB. Markers of innate immune function are associated with vitamin a stores in men. J Nutr. 2009 Feb;139(2):377-85.

Astley SB, Elliott RM. How strong is the evidence that lycopene supplementation can modify biomarkers of oxidative damage and DNA repair in human lymphocytes? J Nutr. 2005 Aug;135(8):2071S-3S.

Astley SB et al. Evidence that dietary supplementation with carotenoids and carotenoid-rich foods modulates the DNA damage: repair balance in human lymphocytes. Br J Nutr. 2004 Jan;91(1):63-72.

Alves LA, de Carvalho AC, Savino W. Gap junctions: a novel route for direct cell-cell communication in the immune system? Immunol Today. 1998 Jun;19(6):269-75.

Ben-Dor A, Steiner M, Gheber L, Danilenko M, Dubi N, Linnewiel K, Zick A, Sharoni Y, Levy J. Carotenoids activate the antioxidant response element transcription system. Mol Cancer Ther. 2005 Jan;4(1).177-86.

Blask DE. Melatonin, sleep disturbance and cancer risk. Sleep Med Rev. 2009 Aug;13(4):257-64.

Boileau TW, Liao Z, Kim S, Lemeshow S, Erdman JW Jr, Clinton SK. Prostate carcinogenesis in N-methyl-N-nitrosourea (NMU)-testosterone-treated rats fed tomato powder, lycopene, or energy-restricted diets. J Natl Cancer Inst. 2003 Nov 5;95(21):1578-86.

Bowen P, Chen L, Stacewicz-Sapuntzakis M, Duncan C, Sharifi R, Ghosh L et al. Tomato sauce supplementation and prostate cancer: lycopene accumulation and modulation of biomarkers of carcinogenesis. Exp Biol Med (Maywood). 2002 Nov;227(10):886-93.

Bravi F, Bosetti C, Dal Maso L et al .Food groups and risk of benign prostatic hyperplasia. Urology. 2006 Jan;67(1):73-9.

Büchner FL, Bueno-de-Mesquita HB, Linseisen J, Boshuizen HC, Kiemeney LA, Ros MM, Overvad K et al. Fruits and vegetables consumption and the risk of histological subtypes of lung cancer in the European Prospective Investigation into Cancer and Nutrition (EPIC). Cancer Causes Control. 2010 Mar;21(3):357-71.

Caple F, Williams EA, Spiers A, Tyson J, Burtle B, Daly AK, Mathers JC, Hesketh JE.Inter-individual variation in DNA damage and base excision repair in young, healthy non-smokers: effects of dietary supplementation and genotype. Br J Nutr. 2010 Jun;103(11):1585-93.

Chalabi N, Delort L, Le Corre L, Satih S, Bignon YJ, Bernard-Gallon D. Gene signature of breast cancer cell lines treated with lycopene. Pharmacogenomics. 2006 Jul;7(5):663-72.

Chan JM, Holick CN, Leitzmann MF, Rimm EB, Willett WC, Stampfer MJ, Giovannucci EL. Diet after diagnosis and the risk of prostate cancer progression, recurrence, and death (United States). Cancer Causes Control. 2006 Mar;17(2):199-208.

Chew BP, Park JS. Carotenoid action on the immune response. J Nutr. 2004 Jan;134(1):257S-261S.

Chew BP, Brown CM, Park JS, Mixter PF. Dietary lutein inhibits mouse mammary tumor growth by regulating angiogenesis and apoptosis. Anticancer Res. 2003 Jul-Aug;23(4):3333-9.

Cho S, Lee DH, Won CH, Kim SM, Lee S, Lee MJ, Chung JH. Differential effects of low-dose and high-dose beta-carotene supplementation on the signs of photoaging and type I procollagen gene expression in human skin in vivo. Dermatology. 2010;221(2):160-71.

Collins AR. Antioxidant intervention as a route to cancer prevention. Eur J Cancer. 2005;41(13):1923-30.

Cui Y, Shikany JM, Liu S, Shagufta Y, Rohan TE. Selected antioxidants and risk of hormone receptor-defined invasive breast cancers among postmenopausal women in the Women's Health Initiative Observational Study. Am Clin Nutr. 2008 Apr;87(4):1009-18.

Dahiya K, Dhankhar R, Madaan H, Singh V, Arora K. Nitric oxide and antioxidant status in head and neck carcinoma before and after radiotherapy. Ann Clin Lab Sci. 2012 Winter;42(1):94-7.

DeGroff VL, Clinton SK. A combination of tomato and soy products for men with recurring prostate cancer and rising prostate specific antigen. Nutr Cancer. 2008;60(2):145-54.

Di Mascio P, Kaiser S, Sies H. Lycopene as the most efficient biological carotenoid singlet oxygen quencher. Arch Biochem Biophys. 1989 Nov 1;274(2):532-8.

Endogenous Hormones and Breast Cancer Collaborative Group, Key TJ, Appleby PN, Reeves GK, Roddam AW. Insulin-like growth factor 1 (IGF1), IGF binding protein 3 (IGFBP3), and breast cancer risk: pooled individual data analysis of 17 prospective studies. Lancet Oncol. 2010 Jun;11(6):530-42.

Friedlander PL. Genomic instability in head and neck cancer patients. Head Neck. 2001 Aug;23(8):683-91.

Gonzalez CA, Riboli E. Diet and cancer prevention: Contributions from the European Prospective Investigation into Cancer and Nutrition (EPIC) study. Eur J Cancer. 2010 Sep;46(14):2555-62.

Giovannucci E. A review of epidemiologic studies of tomatoes, lycopene, and prostate cancer. *Exp. Biol. Med. (Maywood)* 2002;227:852–859.

Giovannucci E, Ascherio A, Rimm EB, Stampfer MJ, Colditz GA, Willett WC. Intake of carotenoids and retinol in relation to risk of prostate cancer. J Natl Cancer Inst. 1995 Dec 6;87(23):1767-76.

Gonzalez CA, Riboli E. Diet and cancer prevention: Contributions from the European Prospective Investigation into Cancer and Nutrition (EPIC) study. Eur J Cancer. 2010 Sep;46(14):2555-62.

Grainger EM, Schwartz SJ, Wang S, et al. A combination of tomato and soy products for men with recurring prostate cancer and rising prostate specific antigen. Nutr Cancer. 2008 Mar-Apr;60(2):145-54.

Graydon R, Gilchrist SE, Young IS, Obermüller-Jevic U, Hasselwander O, Woodside JV. Effect of lycopene supplementation on insulin-like growth factor-1 and insulin-like growth factor binding protein-3: a double-blind, placebo-controlled trial. Eur J Clin Nutr. 2007 Oct;61(10):1196-200.

Hughes DA. Carotenoids. IN: Hughes DA, Bendich A, Darlingtoin LG (Eds). *Diet and Human Immune Function*. New Jersey: Human Press, 2004.

Hwang ES, Bowen PE. Can the consumption of tomatoes or lycopene reduce cancer risk? Integr Cancer Ther. 2002 Jun;1(2):121-32.

Jatoi A, Burch P, Hillman D, Vanyo JM, Dakhil S, Nikcevich D, Rowland K, Morton R, Flynn PJ, Young C, Tan W; North Central Cancer Treatment Group. A tomato-based, lycopene-containing intervention for androgen-independent prostate cancer: results of a Phase II study from the North Central Cancer Treatment Group. Urology. 2007 Feb;69(2):289-94.

Kabat GC, Kim M, Adams-Campbell LL et al. Longitudinal study of serum carotenoid, retinol, and tocopherol concentrations in relation to breast cancer risk among postmenopausal women. Am J Clin Nutr. 2009 Jul;90:162-9.

Karaman E, Uzun H, Papila I et al. Serum paraoxonase activity and oxidative DNA damage in patients with laryngeal squamous cell carcinoma. J Craniofac Surg. 2010 Nov;21(6):1745-9.

Kavanaugh CJ, Trumbo PR, Ellwood KC. The U.S. Food and Drug Administration's evidence-based review for qualified health claims: tomatoes, lycopene, and cancer. J Natl Cancer Inst. 2007 Jul 18;99(14):1074-85.

Key TJ. Fruit and vegetables and cancer risk. Br J Cancer. 2011 Jan 4;104(1):6-11.

Key TJ, Appleby PN, Allen NE et al. Plasma carotenoids, retinol, and tocopherols and the risk of prostate cancer in the European Prospective Investigation into Cancer and Nutrition study. Am J Clin Nutr. 2007 Sep;86(3):672-81.

Kristal AR, Arnold KB, Schenk JM et al. Dietary patterns, supplement use, and the risk of symptomatic benign prostatic hyperplasia: results from the prostate cancer prevention trial. Am J Epidemiol. 2008;167:925-34.

Lorenzo Y, Azqueta A, Luna L, Bonilla F, Domínguez G, Collins AR. The carotenoid beta-cryptoxanthin stimulates the repair of DNA oxidation damage in addition to acting as an antioxidant in human cells. Carcinogenesis. 2009 Feb;30(2):308-14.

McEligot AJ, Largent J, Ziogas A, Peel D, Anton-Culver H.Dietary fat, fiber, vegetable, and micronutrients are associated with overall survival in postmenopausal women diagnosed with breast cancer. Nutr Cancer. 2006;55(2):132-40.

Mignone LI, Giovannucci E, Newcomb PA et al. Dietary carotenoids and the risk of invasive breast cancer. Int Cancer. 2009 Jun 15;124(12):2929-37.

Miller AB, Altenburg HP, Bueno–de–Mesquita B, et al. Fruits and vegetables and lung cancer: Findings from the European Prospective Investigation into Cancer and Nutrition. Int J Cancer. 2004;108:269–276.

Mohanty NK, Saxena S, Singh UP, Goyal NK, Arora RP. Lycopene as a chemopreventive agent in the treatment of high-grade prostate intraepithelial neoplasia. Urol Oncol. 2005 Nov-Dec;23(6):383-5.

Molnár J, Engi H, Hohmann J et al. Reversal of multidrug resitance by natural substances from plants. Curr Top Med Chem. 2010;10(17):1757-68.

Nahum A, Hirsch K, Danilenko M, Watts CK, Prall OW, Levy J, Sharoni Y. Lycopene inhibition of cell cycle progression in breast and endometrial cancer cells is associated with reduction in cyclin D levels and retention of p27(Kip1) in the cyclin E-cdk2 complexes. Oncogene. 2001 Jun 7;20(26):3428-36.

Obermüller-Jevic UC, Hellmis E, Koch W, Jacobi G, Biesalski HK. Lycopene inhibits disease progression in patients with benign prostate hyperplasia. Schwarz S,.J Nutr. 2008 Jan;138(1):49-53.

Pool-Zobel BL et al. Mechanisms by which vegetable consumption reduces genetic damage in humans. Cancer Epidemiol Biomarkers Prev. 1998 Oct;7(10):891-9.

Psaltopoulou T, Kosti RI, Haidopoulos D, Dimopoulos M, Panagiotakos DB. Olive oil intake is inversely related to cancer prevalence: a systematic review and a meta-analysis of 13,800 patients and 23,340 controls in 19 observational studies. Lipids Health Dis. 2011 Jul 30;10:127.

Rao AV, Fleshner N, Agarwal S. Serum and tissue lycopene and biomarkers of oxidation in prostate cancer patients: a case-control study. Nutr Cancer 1999; 33:159-64.

Reedy J, Wirfält E, Flood A, Mitrou PN, Krebs-Smith SM, Kipnis V, Midthune D et al. Comparing 3 dietary pattern methods--cluster analysis, factor analysis, and index analysis--With colorectal cancer risk: The NIH-AARP Diet and Health Study. Am J Epidemiol. 2010 Feb 15;171(4):479-87.

Rock CL, Natarajan L, Pu M et al. Longitudinal biological exposure to carotenoids is associated with breast cancer-free survival in the Women's Healthy Eating and Living Study. Cancer Epidemiol Biomarkers Prev. 2009 Feb;18(2):486-94

Rock CL, Flatt SW, Natarajan L et al. Plasma carotenoids and recurrence-free survival in women with a history of breast cancer. J Clin Oncol. 2005 Sep 20;23(27):6631-8.

Rosenzweig SA, Atreya HS. Defining the pathway to insulin-like growth factor system targeting in cancer. Biochem Pharmacol. 2010 Oct 15;80(8):1115-24.

Sakhi AK, Russnes KM, Thoresen M, Bastani NE, Karlsen A, Smeland S, Blomhoff R. Pre-radiotherapy plasma carotenoids and markers of oxidative stress are associated with survival in head and neck squamous cell carcinoma patients: a prospective study. BMC Cancer. 2009 Dec 21;9:458.

Scandalios JG. Oxidative stress: molecular perception and transduction of signals triggering antioxidant gene defenses. Braz J Med Biol Res. 2005 Jul;38(7):995-1014.

Schwarz S, Obermüller-Jevic UC, Hellmis E, Koch W, Jacobi G, Biesalski HK Lycopene inhibits disease progression in patients with benign prostate hyperplasia. J Nutr. 2008 Jan;138(1):49-53.

Sharoni Y, Agbaria R, Amir H, Ben-Dor A, Bobilev I, Doubi N, Giat Y, et al. Modulation of transcriptional activity by antioxidant carotenoids. Mol Aspects Med. 2003 Dec;24(6):371-84.

Sharoni Y, Danilenko M, Dubi N, Ben-Dor A, Levy J. Carotenoids and transcription. Arch Biochem Biophys. 2004 Oct 1;430(1):89-96.

Soulitzis N, Karyotis I, Delakas D, Spandidos DA. Expression analysis of peptide growth factors VEGF, FGF2, TGFB1, EGF and IGF1 in prostate cancer and benign prostatic hyperplasia. Int J Oncol. 2006 Aug;29:305-14.

Tamimi RM, Colditz GA, Hankinson SE. Circulating carotenoids, mammographic density, and subsequent risk of breast cancer. Cancer Res. 2009 Dec 15;69(24):9323-9.

van Breemen RB, Pajkovic N. Multitargeted therapy of cancer by lycopene. Cancer Lett. 2008; 8;269:339-51.

Veglia F, Matullo G, Vineis P. Bulky DNA adducts and risk of cancer: a meta-analysis. Cancer Epidemiol Biomarkers Prev. 2003 Feb;12(2):157-60.

Veprik A, Khanin M, Linnewiel Hermoni K, Danilenko M, Levy Y, Sharoni Y. Polyphenols, isothiocyanates and carotenoid derivatives enhance estrogenic activity in bone cells but inhibit it in breast cancer cells. Am J Physiol Endocrinol Metab. 2011 Aug 30. doi:10.1152/ajpendo.00142.2011.

Vrieling A, Voskuil DW, Bonfrer JM et al. Lycopene supplementation elevates circulating insulin-like growth factor binding protein-1 and -2 concentrations in persons at greater risk of colorectal cancer. Am J Clin Nutr. 2007 Nov;86(5):1456-62.

Walfisch S, Walfisch Y, Kirilov E et al. Tomato lycopene extract supplementation decreases insulin-like growth factor-1 levels in colon cancer patients. Eur J Cancer Prev. 2007 Aug;16(4):298-303.

Watzl B, Bub A, Brandstetter BR, Rechkemmer G. Modulation of human T-lymphocyte functions by the consumption of carotenoid-rich vegetables. Br J Nutr. 1999 Nov;82(5):383-9.

Watzl B, Bub A, Briviba K, Rechkemmer G. Supplementation of a low-carotenoid diet with tomato or carrot juice modulates immune functions in healthy men. Ann Nutr Metab. 2003;47(6):255-61.

References: Chapter Five: Crucifers Against Cancer

Ahn J, Gammon MD, Santella RM et al. Effects of glutathione S-transferase A1 (GSTA1) genotype and potential modifiers on breast cancer risk. Carcinogenesis. 2006 Sep;27(9):1876-82.

Ambrosone CB, McCann SE, Freudenheim JL, Marshall JR, Zhang Y, Shields PG. Breast cancer risk in premenopausal women is inversely associated with consumption of broccoli, a source of isothiocyanates, but is not modified by GST genotype. J Nutr. 2004 May;134(5):1134-8.

Aubertin-Leheudre M, Gorbach S, Woods M, Dwyer JT, Goldin B, Adlercreutz H. Fat/fiber intakes and sex hormones in healthy premenopausal women in USA. J Steroid Biochem Mol Biol. 2008 Nov;112(1-3):32-9.

Aune D, Chan DS, Vieira AR, Navarro Rosenblatt DA, Vieira R, Greenwood DC, Norat T. Dietary compared with blood concentrations of carotenoids and breast cancer risk: a systematic review and meta-analysis of prospective studies. Am J Clin Nutr. 2012 Jul 3. [Epub ahead of print]

Aune D, Chan DS, Vieira AR, Navarro Rosenblatt DA, Vieira R, Greenwood DC, Norat T. Fruits, vegetables and breast cancer risk: a systematic review and meta-analysis of prospective studies. Breast Cancer Res Treat. 2012 Jun 16. [Epub ahead of print]

Bobe G, Albert PS, Sansbury LB, Lanza E, Schatzkin A, Colburn NH, Cross AJ. Interleukin-6 as a potential indicator for prevention of high-risk adenoma recurrence by dietary flavonols in the polyp prevention trial. Cancer Prev Res (Phila). 2010 Jun;3(6):764-75.

Bobe G, Sansbury LB, Albert PS, Cross AJ, Kahle L, Ashby J, Slattery ML et al. Dietary flavonoids and colorectal adenoma recurrence in the Polyp Prevention Trial. Cancer Epidemiol Biomarkers Prev. 2008 Jun;17(6):1344-53.

Bobe G, Weinstein SJ, Albanes D, Hirvonen T, Ashby J, Taylor PR, Virtamo J, Stolzenberg-Solomon RZ. Flavonoid intake and risk of pancreatic cancer in male smokers (Finland). Cancer Epidemiol Biomarkers Prev. 2008 Mar;17(3):553-62.

Brennan P, Hsu CC, Moullan N et al. Effect of cruciferous vegetables on lung cancer in patients stratified by genetic status: a mendelian randomisation approach. Lancet. 2005 Oct 29-Nov 4;366(9496):1558-60.

Carpenter CL, Yu MC, London SJ. Dietary isothiocyanates, glutathione S-transferase M1 (GSTM1), and lung cancer risk in African Americans and Caucasians from Los Angeles County, California. Nutr Cancer. 2009;61(4):492-9.

Cheung KL, Kong AN. Molecular targets of dietary phenethyl isothiocyanate and sulforaphane for cancer chemoprevention. AAPS J. 2010 Mar;12(1):87-97.

Chen X, Danes C, Lowe M, Herliczek TW, Keyomarsi K. Activation of the estrogen-signaling pathway by p21(WAF1/CIP1) in estrogen receptor-negative breast cancer cells. J Natl Cancer Inst. 2000 Sep 6;92:1403-13.

Choi S, Singh SV. Bax and bak are required for apoptosis induction by sulforaphane, a cruciferous vegetable-derived cancer chemopreventive agent. Cancer Res. 2005 Mar 1;65(5):2035-43.

Chyou PH, Nomura AM, Hankin JH, Stemmermann GN. A case-cohort study of diet and stomach cancer. Cancer Res. 1990 Dec 1;50(23):7501-4.

Cohen JH, Kristal AR, Stanford JL. Fruit and vegetable intakes and prostate cancer risk. J Natl Cancer Inst. 2000 ;92:61-8.

Fimognari C, Nusse M, Berti F, Iori R, Cantelli-Forti G, Hrelia P. Sulforaphane modulates cell cycle and apoptosis in transformed and non-transformed human T lymphocytes. Ann N Y Acad Sci. 2003 Dec;1010:393-8.

Gaudet MM, Olshan AF, Poole C, Weissler MC, Watson M, Bell DA. Diet, GSTM1 and GSTT1 and head and neck cancer. Carcinogenesis. 2004 May;25(5):735-40.

Gold B, Kalush F, Bergeron J, Scott K et al. Estrogen receptor genotypes and haplotypes associated with breast cancer risk. Cancer Res. 2004 Dec 15;64(24):8891-900.

Hara M, Hanaoka T, Kobayashi M et al.. Cruciferous vegetables, mushrooms, and gastrointestinal cancer risks in a multicenter, hospital-based case-control study in Japan. Nutr Cancer. 2003;46(2):138-47.

Haristoy X, Angioi-Duprez K, Duprez A, Lozniewski A. Efficacy of sulforaphane in eradicating Helicobacter pylori in human gastric xenografts implanted in nude mice. Antimicrob Agents Chemother. 2003;47:3982-4.

Hiipakka RA, Zhang HZ, Dai W, Dai Q, Liao S. Structure-activity relationships for inhibition of human 5alpha reductases by polyphenols. Biochem Pharmacol. 2002 Mar 15;63(6):1165-76.

Joseph MA, Moysich KB, Freudenheim JL, Shields PG, Bowman ED, Zhang Y, Marshall JR, Ambrosone CB. Cruciferous vegetables, genetic polymorphisms in glutathione S-transferases M1 and T1, and prostate cancer risk. Nutr Cancer. 2004;50(2):206-13.

Kall MA, Vang O, Clausen J. Effects of dietary broccoli on human in vivo drug metabolizing enzymes: evaluation of caffeine, oestrone and chlorzoxazone metabolism. Carcinogenesis. 1996 Apr;17(4):793-9.

Keck AS, Finley JW. Cruciferous vegetables: cancer protective mechanisms of glucosinolate hydrolysis products and selenium. Integr Cancer Ther. 2004 Mar;3(1):5-12.

Kolonel LN, Hankin JH, Whittemore AS, Wu AH, Gallagher RP, Wilkens LR et al. Vegetables, fruits, legumes and prostate cancer: a multiethnic case-control study. Cancer Epidemiol Biomarkers Prev. 2000;9:795-804.

Kirsh VA, Peters U, Mayne ST, Subar AF, Chatterjee N, Johnson CC, Hayes RB; Prostate, Lung, Colorectal and Ovarian Cancer Screening Trial. Prospective study of fruit and vegetable intake and risk of prostate cancer. J Natl Cancer Inst. 2007 Aug 1;99(15):1200-9.

Lampe JW. Interindividual differences in response to plant-based diets: implications for cancer risk. Am J Clin Nutr. 2009 May;89(5):1553S-1557S.

Lee SA, Fowke JH, Lu W, Ye C, Zheng Y, Cai Q, Gu K, Gao YT, Shu XO, Zheng W. Cruciferous vegetables, the GSTP1 Ile105Val genetic polymorphism, and breast cancer risk. Am J Clin Nutr. 2008 Mar;87(3):753-60.

Lewis-Wambi JS, Jordan VC. Estrogen regulation of apoptosis: how can one hormone stimulate and inhibit? Breast Cancer Res. 2009;11(3):206

Mandlekar S, Yu R, Tan TH, Kong AN. Activation of caspase-3 and c-Jun NH2-terminal kinase-1 signaling pathways in tamoxifen-induced apoptosis of human breast cancer cells. Cancer Res. 2000;60(21):5995-6000.

Loo G. Redox-sensitive mechanisms of phytochemical-mediated inhibition of cancer cell proliferation (review). J Nutr Biochem. 2003 Feb;14(2):64-73.

McQuillan GM, Kruszon-Moran D, Kottiri BJ, Curtin LR, Lucas JW, Kington RS. Racial and ethnic differences in the seroprevalence of 6 infectious diseases in the United States: data from NHANES III, 1988-1994. Am J Public Health. 2004 Nov;94(11):1952-8.

Melchini A, Costa C, Traka M, Miceli N, Mithen R, De Pasquale R, Trovato A. Erucin, a new promising cancer chemopreventive agent from rocket salads, shows anti-proliferative activity on human lung carcinoma A549 cells. Food Chem Toxicol. 2009 Jul;47(7):1430-6.

Miller K. Estrogen and DNA damage: the silent source of breast cancer? J Natl Cancer Inst. 2003;95(2):100-102.

Moy KA, Yuan JM, Chung FL, Wang XL, Van Den Berg D, Wang R, Gao YT, Yu MC.Isothiocyanates, glutathione S-transferase M1 and T1 polymorphisms and gastric cancer risk: a prospective study of men in Shanghai, China. Int J Cancer. 2009 Dec 1;125(11):2652-9.

Moore LE, Brennan P, Karami S, Hung RJ, Hsu C, Boffetta P, Toro J et al. Glutathione S-transferase polymorphisms, cruciferous vegetable intake and cancer risk in the Central and Eastern European Kidney Cancer Study. Carcinogenesis. 2007 Sep;28(9):1960-4.

Nöthlings U, Murphy SP, Wilkens LR, Henderson BE, Kolonel LN.Flavonols and pancreatic cancer risk: the multiethnic cohort study. Am J Epidemiol. 2007 Oct 15;166(8):924-31.

Sansbury LB, Wanke K, Albert PS, Kahle L, Schatzkin A, Lanza E; Polyp Prevention Trial Study Group. The effect of strict adherence to a high-fiber, high-fruit and -vegetable, and low-fat eating pattern on adenoma recurrence. Am J Epidemiol. 2009 Sep 1;170(5):576-84.

Schatzkin A, Park Y, Leitzmann MF, Hollenbeck AR, Cross AJ. Prospective study of dietary fiber, whole grain foods, and small intestinal cancer. Gastroenterology. 2008 Oct;135(4):1163-7.

Seow A, Yuan JM, Sun CL, Van Den Berg D, Lee HP, Yu MC. Dietary isothiocyanates, glutathione S-transferase polymorphisms and colorectal cancer risk in the Singapore Chinese Health Study. Carcinogenesis. 2002 Dec;23(12):2055-61.

Steinbrecher A, Nimptsch K, Hüsing A, Rohrmann S, Linseisen J. Dietary glucosinolate intake and risk of prostate cancer in the EPIC-Heidelberg cohort study. Int J Cancer. 2009 Nov 1;125(9):2179-86.

Talalay P, Dinkova-Kostova AT, Holtzclaw WD. Importance of phase 2 gene regulation in protection against e electrophile and reactive oxygen toxicity and carcinogenesis. Adv Enzyme Regul. 2003;43:121-34.

Tang L, Zirpoli GR, Guru K, Moysich KB, Zhang Y, Ambrosone CB, McCann SE. Consumption of raw cruciferous vegetables is inversely associated with bladder cancer risk. Cancer Epidemiol Biomarkers Prev. 2008 Apr;17(4):938-44.

Traka M, Gasper AV, Melchini A et al. Broccoli consumption interacts with GSTM1 to perturb oncogenic signaling pathways in the prostate. PLoS ONE. 2008 Jul 2;3(7):e2568.

van Houten ME, Gooren LJ. Differences in reproductive endocrinology between Asian men and Caucasian men--a literature review. Asian J Androl. 2000 Mar;2(1):13-20.

Wang L, Liu D, Ahmed T, Chung FL, Conaway C, Chiao JW. Targeting cell cycle machinery as a molecular mechanism of sulforaphane in prostate cancer prevention. Int J Oncol. 2004 Jan;24(1):187-92.

Xiao D, Johnson CS, Trump DL, Singh SV. Proteasome-mediated degradation of cell division cycle 25C and cyclin-dependent kinase 1 in phenethyl isothiocyanate-induced G2-M-phase cell cycle arrest in PC-3 human prostate cancer cells. Mol Cancer Ther. 2004 May;3(5):567-75.

Yang G, Gao YT, Shu XO, Cai Q, Li GL, Li HL, Ji BT, Rothman N, Dyba M, Xiang YB, Chung FL, Chow WH, Zheng W. Isothiocyanate exposure, glutathione S-transferase polymorphisms, and colorectal cancer risk. Am J Clin Nutr. 2010 Mar;91(3):704-11.

References: Chapter Six: Spice it Up: Add Flavor, Subtract Cancer Risk

Abdullah TH, Kandil O, Elkadi A, Carter J. Garlic revisited: therapeutic for the major diseases of our times? J Natl Med Assoc. 1988 Apr;80(4):439-45.

Ceschi M, Gutzwiller F, Moch H, Eichholzer M, Probst-Hensch NM. Epidemiology and pathophysiology of obesity as cause of cancer. Swiss Med Wkly. 2007 Jan 27;137(3-4):50-6.

Cryer B. NSAID-Associated Deaths: The Rise and Fall of NSAID-Associated GI Mortality. The American Journal of Gastroenterology (2005) 100, 1694–1695.

Epelbaum R, Schaffer M, Vizel B, Badmaev V, Bar-Sela G. Curcumin and gemcitabine in patients with advanced pancreatic cancer. Nutr Cancer. 2010;62(8):1137-41.

Federico A, Morgillo F, Tuccillo C, Ciardiello F, Loguercio C. Chronic inflammation and oxidative stress in human carcinogenesis. Int J Cancer 2007 Dec 1;121(11):2381-6.

González-Pérez A, García Rodríguez LA, López-Ridaura R. Effects of non-steroidal anti-inflammatory drugs on cancer sites other than the colon and rectum: a meta-analysis. BMC Cancer. 2003 Oct 3;3:28.

Hartnett L, Egan LJ. Inflammation, DNA methylation and colitis-associated cancer. Carcinogenesis. 2012 Apr;33(4):723-31.

Harris RE. Cyclooxygenase-2 (cox-2) and the inflammogenesis of cancer. Subcell Biochem. 2007;42:93-126.

He ZY, Shi CB, Wen H, Li FL, Wang BL, Wang J. Upregulation of p53 expression in patients with colorectal cancer by administration of curcumin. Cancer Invest. 2011 Mar;29(3):208-13.

Hedlund M, Padler-Karavani V, Varki NM, Varki A. Evidence for a human-specific mechanism for diet and antibody-mediated inflammation in carcinoma progression. Proc Natl Acad Sci U S A. 2008; 105:18936-41.

Kunnumakkar AB, Anand P, Aggarwal BB. Curcumin inhibits proliferation, invasion, angiogenesis and metastasis of different cancers through interaction with multiple cell signaling proteins. Cancer Letters 2008; 269:199–225.

Lin JK. Suppression of protein kinase C and nuclear oncogene expression as possible action mechanisms of cancer chemoprevention by curcumin. Arch Pharm Res. 2004 Jul; 27(7):683-92.

Howard EW, Lee DT, Chiu YT, Chua CW, Wang X, Wong YC. Evidence of a novel docetaxel sensitizer, garlic-derived S-allylmercaptocysteine, as a treatment option for hormone refractory prostate cancer. Int J Cancer. 2008 May 1;122(9):1941-8.

Ide N, Lau BH. Garlic compounds minimize intracellular oxidative stress and inhibit nuclear factor-kappa b activation. J Nutr. 2001 Mar;131(3s):1020S-6S.

Kim JY, Kwon O. Garlic intake and cancer risk: an analysis using the Food and Drug Administration's evidence-based review system for the scientific evaluation of health claims. Am J Clin Nutr. 2009 Jan;89(1):257-64.

Lamm DL, Riggs DR. Enhanced immunocompetence by garlic: role in bladder cancer and other malignancies. J Nutr. 2001 Mar;131(3s):1067S-70S.

Loizou GD, Cocker J. The effects of alcohol and diallyl sulphide on CYP2E1 activity in humans: a phenotyping study using chlorzoxazone. Hum Exp Toxicol. 2001 Jul;20(7):321-7.

Mahmud S, Franco E, Aprikian A. Prostate cancer and use of nonsteroidal anti-inflammatory drugs: systematic review and meta-analysis. Br J Cancer. 2004 Jan 12;90(1):93-9.

Mirunalini S, Arulmozhi V, Arulmozhi T. Curative Effect of Garlic on Alcoholic Liver Diseased Patients. Jordan Journal of Biological Sciences 2010; 3(4): 147-152.

Nagini S. Cancer chemoprevention by garlic and its organosulfur compounds-panacea or promise? Anticancer Agents Med Chem. 2008 Apr;8(3):313-21.

Olsen JH, Friis S Poulsen AH, et al. Use of NSAIDs, smoking and lung cancer risk.. Br J Cancer. 2008 Jan 15;98(1):232-7.

Pelucchi C, Tramacere I, Boffetta P, Negri E, La Vecchia C. Alcohol consumption and cancer risk. Nutr Cancer. 2011;63(7):983-90.

Rothwell PM, Price JF, Fowkes FG et al. Short-term effects of daily aspirin on cancer incidence, mortality, and non-vascular death: analysis of the time course of risks and benefits in 51 randomised controlled trials. Lancet. 2012 Apr 28;379(9826):1602-12.

Salem S, Salahi M, Mohseni M, Ahmadi H, Mehrsai A, Jahani Y, Pourmand G. Major dietary factors and prostate cancer risk: a prospective multicenter case-control study. Nutr Cancer. 2011;63(1):21-7.

Surh YJ. Anti-tumor promoting potential of selected spice ingredients with antioxidative and anti-inflammatory activities: a short review. Food Chem Toxicol. 2002 Aug;40(8):1091-7.

Takkouche B, Regueira-Méndez C, Etminan M. Breast cancer and use of nonsteroidal anti-inflammatory drugs: a meta-analysis. J Natl Cancer Inst. 2008 Oct 15;100(20):1439-47.

Tanaka S, Haruma K, Kunihiro M et al. Effects of aged garlic extract (AGE) on colorectal adenomas: a double-blinded study. Hiroshima J Med Sci. 2004 Dec;53(3-4):39-45.

Tanaka S, Haruma K, Yoshihara M et al. Aged garlic extract has potential suppressive effect on colorectal adenomas in humans. J Nutr. 2006 Mar;136(3 Suppl):821S-826S.

Wang WH, Huang JQ, Zheng GF, Lam SK, Karlberg J, Wong BC. Non-steroidal anti-inflammatory drug use and the risk of gastric cancer: a systematic review and meta-analysis. J Natl Cancer Inst. 2003 Dec 3;95(23):1784-91.

Wu G, Fang YZ, Yang S, Lupton JR, Turner ND. Glutathione metabolism and its implications for health. J Nutr. 2004 Mar;134(3):489-92.

Zhou Y, Zhuang W, Hu W, Liu GJ, Wu TX, Wu XT. Consumption of large amounts of Allium vegetables reduces risk for gastric cancer in a meta-analysis. Gastroenterology. 2011 Jul;141(1):80-9.

References: Chapter Seven: A grape way to reduce cancer risk

Aziz MH, Afaq F, Ahmad N. Prevention of ultraviolet-B radiation damage by resveratrol in mouse skin is mediated via modulation in survivin. Photchem Photobiol 2005; 81:25-31.

Bagnardi V, Blangiardo M, La Vecchia C, Corrao G. Alcohol consumption and the risk of cancer: a meta-analysis. Alcohol Res Health. 2001;25(4):263-70.

Baliunas DO, Taylor BJ, Irving H, Roerecke M, Patra J, Mohapatra S, Rehm J. Alcohol as a risk factor for type 2 diabetes: A systematic review and meta-analysis. Diabetes Care. 2009 Nov;32(11):2123-32.

Baur JA, Sinclair DA. Therapeutic potential of resveratrol: the in vivo evidence. Nat Rev Drug Discov. 2006 5:493-506.

Bianchini F, Vainio H. Wine and resveratrol: mechanisms of cancer prevention? Eur J Cancer Prev. 2003 Oct; 12(5):417-25.

Boffetta P, Hashibe M. Alcohol and cancer. Lancet Oncol. 2006 Feb;7(2):149-56.

Brown VA, Patel KR, Viskaduraki M et al. Repeat dose study of the cancer chemopreventive agent resveratrol in healthy volunteers: safety, pharmacokinetics, and effect on the insulin-like growth factor axis. Cancer Res. 2010 Nov 15;70(22):9003-11.

Burns J, Yokota T, Ashihara H, Lean ME, Crozier A. Plant foods and herbal sources of resveratrol. J Agric Food Chem. 2002 May 22;50(11):3337-40.

Chao C. Associations between beer, wine, and liquor consumption and lung cancer risk: a meta-analysis. Cancer Epidemiol Biomarkers Prev. 2007 Nov;16(11):2436-47.

Chao C, Slezak JM, Caan BJ, Quinn VP. Alcoholic beverage intake and risk of lung cancer: the California Men's Health Study. Cancer Epidemiol Biomarkers Prev. 2008 Oct;17(10):2692-9.

Chiu BC, Cerhan JR, Gapstur SM et al. Alcohol consumption and non-Hodgkin lymphoma in a cohort of older women. Br J Cancer. 1999; 80(9):1476-82.

Chow HH, Garland LL, Hsu CH et al. Resveratrol modulates drug- and carcinogen-metabolizing enzymes in a healthy volunteer study. Cancer Prev Res (Phila). 2010 Sep;3(9):1168-75.

Collins MA, Neafsey EJ, Mukamal KJ, Gray MO, Parks DA, Das DK, Korthuis RJ. Alcohol in moderation, cardioprotection, and neuroprotection: epidemiological considerations and mechanistic studies. Alcohol Clin Exp Res. 2009 Feb;33(2):206-19.

Couto E, Boffetta P, Lagiou P et al. Mediterranean dietary pattern and cancer risk in the EPIC cohort. Br J Cancer. 2011 Apr 26;104(9):1493-9.

Eng ET, Williams D, Mandava U, Kirma M, Tekmal RR, Chen S. Anti-aromatase chemicals in red wine. Ann N Y Acad Sci. 2002 Jun;963:239-46.

Fung TT, Hunter DJ, Spiegelman D, Colditz GA, Rimm EB, Willett WC. Intake of alcohol and alcoholic beverages and the risk of basal cell carcinoma of the skin.Cancer Epidemiol Biomarkers Prev. 2002 Oct;11(10 Pt 1):1119-22.

Giovannucci E, Harlan DM, Archer MC et al. Diabetes and Cancer: A Consensus Report. CA Cancer J Clin 2010;60:207-221.

Goodman MT, Tung KH. Alcohol consumption and the risk of borderline and invasive ovarian cancer. Obstet Gynecol. 2003 Jun;101(6):1221-8.

Gresele P, Pignatelli P, Guglielmini G et al. Resveratrol, at concentrations attainable with moderate wine consumption, stimulates human platelet nitric oxide production. J Nutr. 2008 Sep;138(9):1602-8.

Kaneuchi M, Sasaki M, Tanaka Y, Yamamoto R, Sakuragi N, Dahiya R. Resveratrol suppresses growth of Ishikawa cells through down-regulation of EGF. Int J Oncol. 2003 Oct;23(4):1167-72.

Khan SI, Zhao J, Khan IA, Walker LA, Dasmahapatra AK. Potential utility of natural products as regulators of breast cancer-associated aromatase promoters. Reprod Biol Endocrinol. 2011 Jun 21;9:91.

Kimura Y, Sumiyoshi M, Baba K. Antitumor activities of synthetic and natural stilbenes through antiangiogenic action. Cancer Sci. 2008 Oct;99(10):2083-96.

Kloner RA, Rezkalla SH. To drink or not to drink? That is the question. Circulation. 2007 Sep 11;116:1306-17.

Kundu JK, Surh YJ. Cancer chemopreventive and therapeutic potential of resveratrol: mechanistic perspectives. Cancer Lett. 2008 Oct 8;269(2):243-61.

Levi F, Pasche C, Lucchini F, Ghidoni R, Ferraroni M, La Vecchia C. Resveratrol and breast cancer risk. Eur J Cancer Prev. 2005 Apr;14(2):139-42.

Mitchell SH, Zhu W, Young CY. Resveratrol inhibits the expression and function of the androgen receptor in LNCaP prostate cancer cells. Cancer Res. 1999 Dec 1;59(23):5892-5.

Opipari AW Jr, Tan L, Boitano AE, Sorenson DR, Aurora A, Liu JR. Resveratrol-induced autophagocytosis in ovarian cancer cells. Cancer Res. 2004 Jan 15;64(2):696-703.

Platz EA, Leitzmann MF, Rimm EB et al. Alcohol intake, drinking patterns, and risk of prostate cancer in a large prospective cohort study. Am J Epidemiol. 2004 Mar 1;159(5):444-53.

Provinciali M, Re F, Donnini A, Orlando F, Bartozzi B, Di Stasio G, Smorlesi A. Effect of resveratrol on the development of spontaneous mammary tumors in HER-2/neu transgenic mice. Int J Cancer 2005; May 20; 115(1):36-45.

Ronksley PE, Brien SE, Turner BJ, Mukamal KJ, Ghali WA. Association of alcohol consumption with selected cardiovascular disease outcomes: a systematic review and meta-analysis. BMJ. 2011 Feb 22;342:d671.

Ruano-Ravina A, Figueiras A, Barros-Dios JM. Type of wine and risk of lung cancer: a case-control study in Spain. Thorax. 2004 Nov;59(11):981-5.

Saleem TS, Basha SD. Red wine: A drink to your heart. J Cardiovasc Dis Res. 2010 Oct;1(4):171-6.

Schoonen WM, Salinas CA, Kiemeney LA, Stanford JL. Alcohol consumption and risk of prostate cancer in middle-aged men. Int J Cancer. 2005 Jan 1;113(1):133-40.

Sofi F, Abbate R, Gensini GF, Casini A. Accruing evidence on benefits of adherence to the Mediterranean diet on health: an updated systematic review and meta-analysis. Am J Clin Nutr. 2010 Nov;92(5):1189-96.

Vachon CM, Kuni CC, Anderson K, Anderson VE, Sellers TA. Association of mammographically defined percent breast density with epidemiologic risk factors for breast cancer (United States). Cancer Causes Control. 2000 Aug;11(7):653-62.

Valenciano A, Henríquez-Hernández LA, Moreno M, Lloret M, Lara PC. Role of IGF-1 Receptor in Radiation Response. Transl Oncol. 2012 Feb;5(1):1-9.

Zamora-Ros R, Andres-Lacueva C, Lamuela-Raventós RM et al. Concentrations of resveratrol and derivatives in foods and estimation of dietary intake in a Spanish population: European Prospective Investigation into Cancer and Nutrition (EPIC)-Spain cohort. Br J Nutr. 2008 Jul;100(1):188-96.

Zatloukal P, Kubik A, Pauk N, Tomasek L, Petruzelka L. Adenocarcinoma of the lung among women: risk associated with smoking, prior lung disease, diet and menstrual and pregnancy history. Lung Cancer. 2003 Sep;41(3):283-93.
Zell JA, McEligot AJ, Ziogas A, Holcombe RF, Anton-Culver H. Differential effects of wine consumption on colorectal cancer outcomes based on family history of the disease. Nutr Cancer. 2007;59(1):36-45.

Chapter Eight: The Grain Gain: How Whole Grains Fight Cancer

Agarwal C, Dhanalakshmi S, Singh RP, Agarwal R. Inositol hexaphosphate inhibits growth and induces G1 arrest and apoptotic death of androgen-dependent human prostate carcinoma LNCaP cells. Neoplasia. 2004 Sep-Oct;6(5):646-59.
Baron JA. Dietary fiber and colorectal cancer: an ongoing saga. JAMA. 2005 Dec 14;294(22):2904-6.
Beyer-Sehlmeyer G, Glei M, Hartmann E et al. Butyrate is only one of several growth inhibitors produced during gut flora-mediated fermentation of dietary fibre sources. Br J Nutr. 2003 Dec;90(6):1057-70.
Daly K, Cuff MA, Fung F, Shirazi-Beechey SP. The importance of colonic butyrate transport to the regulation of genes associated with colonic tissue homeostasis. Biochem Soc Trans. 2005 Aug;33(Pt 4):733-5.
Davie JR. Inhibition of histone deacetylase activity by butyrate. J Nutr. 2003 Jul;133(7 Suppl):2485S-2493S.
Elson CE, Peffley DM, Hentosh P, Mo H. Isoprenoid-mediated inhibition of mevalonate synthesis: potential application to cancer. Proc Soc Exp Biol Med. 1999 Sep;221(4):294-311.
Kasum CM, Jacobs DR Jr, Nicodemus K, Folsom AR. Dietary risk factors for upper aerodigestive tract cancers. Int J Cancer. 2002 May 10;99(2):267-72.
Kautenburger T, Beyer-Sehlmeyer G, Festag G et al. The gut fermentation product butyrate, a chemopreventive agent, suppresses glutathione S-transferase theta (hGSTT1) and cell growth more in human colon adenoma (LT97) than tumor (HT29) cells. J Cancer Res Clin Oncol. 2005 Oct;131(10):692-700.
Klurfeld DM. Dietary fiber-mediated mechanisms in carcinogenesis. Cancer Res. 1992;52(7 Suppl):2055s-59s.
Larsson SC, Giovannucci E, Bergkvist L, Wolk A. Whole grain consumption and risk of colorectal cancer: a population-based cohort of 60,000 women. Br J Cancer. 2005 May 9;92(9):1803-7.
Lupton JR. Microbial degradation products influence colon cancer risk: the butyrate controversy. J Nutr. 2004 Feb;134(2):479-82.
Liu S, Willett WC, Manson JE, Hu FB, Rosner B, Colditz G. Relation between changes in intakes of dietary fiber and grain products and changes in weight and development of obesity among middle-aged women. Am J Clin Nutr. 2003 Nov;78(5):920-7.
Maier JA, Nasulewicz A, Simonacci M, Boninsegna A, Mazur A, Wolf FI. Insights into the mechanisms involved in magnesium-dependent inhibition of primary tumor growth. Nutr Cancer. 2007;59:192-198.
M A M, Pera G, Agudo A, Bueno-de-Mesquita HB et al. Cereal fiber intake may reduce risk of gastric adenocarcinomas: the EPIC-EURGAST study. Int J Cancer 2007; 121(7):1618-23.
Ovesna Z, Vachalkova A, Horvathova K. Taraxasterol and beta-sitosterol: new naturally compounds with chemoprotective/chemopreventive effects. Neoplasma. 2004;51(6):407-14.
Prasad KN, Kumar A, Kochupillai V, Cole WC. High doses of multiple antioxidant vitamins: essential ingredients in improving the efficacy of standard cancer therapy. J Am Coll Nutr. 1999 Feb;18(1):13-25.
Slavin JL. Mechanisms for the impact of whole grain foods on cancer risk. J Am Coll Nutr. 2000 Jun;19(3 Suppl):300S-307S.
Slavin J. Why whole grains are protective: biological mechanisms. Proc Nutr Soc. 2003 Feb;62(1):129-34.
Smeltzer A, Kim YS. The Effects of Bioactive Food Components on p53 Pathway in Cancer Prevention. Nutrition Today 2005; 40(1): 50-53.
von Holtz RL, Fink CS, Awad AB. beta-Sitosterol activates the sphingomyelin cycle and induces apoptosis in LNCaP human prostate cancer cells. Nutr Cancer. 1998;32(1):8-12.
Vucenik I, Shamsuddin AM. Cancer inhibition by inositol hexaphosphate (IP6) and inositol: from laboratory to clinic. J Nutr. 2003 Nov;133(11 Suppl 1):3778S-3784S.
Yin L, Laevsky G, Giardina C. Butyrate suppression of colonocyte NF-kappa B activation and cellular proteasome activity. J Biol Chem. 2001 Nov 30;276(48):44641-6.

INDEX

www.ingramcontent.com/pod-product-compliance
Lightning Source LLC
Chambersburg PA
CBHW051725170526
45167CB00002B/808